Poppy the Street Dog

Poppy the Street Dog

How an extraordinary dog helped bring hope to the homeless

Michelle Clark
with Linda Watson-Brown

SEVEN DIALS

First published in the United Kingdom in 2020 by Seven Dials,
an imprint of The Orion Publishing Group Ltd
Carmelite House, 50 Victoria Embankment,
London EC4Y 0DZ

An Hachette UK company

1 3 5 7 9 10 8 6 4 2

A CIP catalogue record for this book is
available from the British Library.

ISBN (Paperback): 978 1 409 19543 6
ISBN (eBook): 978 1 409 19544 3

Typeset by Born Group

Printed and bound in Great Britain by Clays Ltd, Elcograf S.p.A.

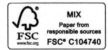

www.orionbooks.co.uk

For Poppy, who made it all happen xx

Poppy

You brought me love, you brought me joy,
You brought me so much light.
It was you who gave me hope, the energy to fight.

I sometimes have to catch my breath,
To know that we're apart.
But you, my darling gorgeous girl,
Are always in my heart.

I truly feel that in our lives,
Our dogs can change all things.
That doesn't change, dear Poppy, now you have your
angel wings.

So, fly my darling, smile your smile,
Run and play and hide.
For one day, someday, I'll be there,
always by your side.

CONTENTS

ONE

This is Me

'Look at this, just look at all of this. It's so beautiful.'

I was speaking to myself, whispering really, but there was someone else there, in spirit, at my side. I felt as if I was looking out at The Sanctuary through the big eyes of the dog who had been with me through so much, but who had crossed over the Rainbow Bridge the year before. I could never have believed that I would be standing here, looking out over three acres, with brightly coloured, luxury kennels behind me, all just waiting for dogs in need. The Sanctuary was well named, not just for those who would benefit from it, but as somewhere that was an incredible symbol for me too. This would be where I could change things, this was where a difference would be made. Looking out over it all, I allowed myself to feel a little bit of pride, even though I knew there was still a long way to go. This wonderful place was finally here, the first steps taken, the foundations well and truly laid, in every sense.

'We've come a long way, Poppy, haven't we, girl?'

Poppy.

The dog who never stopped looking at me, the dog who had inspired all of this. The dog who was no longer here in body, but whose soul was in everything I did.

'You know that this is all down to you, don't you? I miss you so much and I would never have dreamed so big without you.' As I stood there, I felt as if I could almost touch her, as if I could just reach my hand down and scratch behind those ears while she looked up at me with a soppy, doggy smile on her face. If only. There was a hole in my life and my heart without her, and there always would be, but I knew I needed to just concentrate on what was here now, and what would be here in the future.

I'd only met Poppy a few years ago and yet, without her, I wouldn't be standing here gazing at this retreat where street dogs would be brought for care, treatment and rehabilitation. It was a vision come true to have somewhere like this, but it was only one part of my plan to put in place a much bigger structure where those on the streets could access any help they needed, with their beloved dogs beside them every step of the way. None of it would be possible without the inspiration of Poppy. She was the one who had got me here, she was the one who had opened my eyes.

I'm running ahead of myself, as I'd always rather talk about dogs than me, but I'm the one who can give a voice to these animals, so I guess I'd better tell you a few things! I hate attention and I don't really want to chat about anything other than dogs, but it's all part of the story, I suppose. It's the same for all of us, I believe. We can only really tell how we got here when we look back at where we've been.

So, I'm a Londoner through and through and – as you might have guessed by now – I love dogs. I'd say that was enough! I was brought up in the London Borough of Barnet, a city girl who was actually raised with cats rather than dogs. Mum always had a little feline friend around. The first one I remember was Pymmes, a tabby cat who didn't like anyone other than Mum. Mum could get Pymmes to roll over on command, to do all sorts of tricks, but no one else could even make that cat shift an inch across the sofa if she didn't want to. It's not that I wasn't close to her; it was more than she and Mum were in their own little bubble. I can sort of understand it now; I've had so many incredibly close relationships with dogs and cats and adored the times they have been in my life, that I know how important their unconditional love is.

I always loved animals – the fish tank we had with the big silver fat fish called Pharaoh, the ladybirds in the garden that I would put on leaves to keep them safe, the birds that pecked about in the garden – anything at all. Apart from spiders – no to those, thanks very much!

Back then, all the kids went out to play a lot and I kept an eye open for any animals, all the time. I'd have confronted anyone who was cruel to them, so I guess that was my 'animals first' side coming out, even at that young age. Thankfully, I didn't ever have to, but I'm quite sure that they would have known the error of their ways if I'd even had a sniff of animal cruelty. I couldn't understand it then and I can't understand it now. We really don't deserve animals, but we're blessed to have them.

Pymmes was really the only furry creature I had at home though, and I used to write poems about her in English classes at school. However, it was clear that she was really Mum's cat. In fact, Mum was obsessed with cats in general. She'd go to cat sanctuary open days; she'd look out for strays. I'm not sure what she was looking for, but she didn't find it, and she never found another cat that she felt would fit in as well as Pymmes.

Pymmes was definitely the sole owner of us for a while – strictly in line with cats deciding what to do with *us* rather than the other way around!

Pymmes had been with Mum before I came into the picture. Mum had been in a pub one day, and this tiny little lost kitten was brought in. The first thing she did was knock over a bottle of Pimm's, and there was her name – with a little twist – instantly! It must have been love at first sight because Mum brought her back to ours and she settled in immediately, I was told.

When I moved away from home as a teenager, I got a cat of my own whom I called Buster. I was still living in London and had gone to a rescue sanctuary one day, just to look, just to see what sort of kittens they had. I'm not sure anyone could ever walk away from a place like that without taking a little friend home with them, and as soon as I set my eyes on this tiny ball of silvery grey fluff, I immediately fell head over heels.

Having Buster at home was a dream come true. He was great company and I adored nurturing him, as well as finally getting all of the cuddles I had wanted from a pet since I was a little girl. He was mine, all mine, and I'd never had that sense of pure love in my life up until that point. It was then that I came to understand just how perfect animals can be, how they seem to sense what you need, and how they can fill the gaps in your life that you were desperately trying to avoid even looking at.

Buster was a tiny scrap of a thing with specks on his little grey face, and had a really playful nature. I couldn't wait to get back from work every night as he was the best part of my day. He was always so pleased to see me; I never had to go and find him as he would come trotting to my side as soon as I opened the front door. Back then, it was the done thing to give milk to cats as no one really knew that the lactose could cause tummy problems, so Buster always knew that I would pour him a dish when I arrived home. His purring would be like a machine as he wove in and out of my legs, waiting for me to hurry up at the fridge, then contentedly lap at his bowl.

As he grew, I started letting him out. I lived in a quiet cul-de-sac and it would have been cruel to keep him indoors. But, sadly, the inevitable happened and he didn't come home one evening. I searched for him that whole night, finally finding his little body on the side of the road. He had been hit by a car. I was devastated and couldn't even pick him up. I called my mum, barely able to get the words out through my tears. Even though we'd had our moments, she knew what it was to love a cat with all your heart and I could rely on her to help me with this. She took him to the vet, but the poor soul was long gone. He was only two, he'd barely lived any life at all, but it had been full of love, I'd made sure of that.

My heart was breaking but everyone told me it would pass. To some, pets are 'just' that; they are 'just' animals and there can be a sense that it's wrong to mourn them in the same way as a person. When I lost Buster, though, I learned that wasn't the case at all. I actually thought I was abnormal as my grief continued because of the attitude of others. Some people did get terribly upset when their pets passed, of course, but this felt physical as well as emotional to me. My body was heavy – in fact, I thought I could feel the weight of my heart, and there was a constant pressure which I thought would never leave. While some people did treat their pets as family, they didn't seem to look on them as their babies as such. It was different with Buster – he had been my whole world.

I'd connected so strongly with him and now he was gone. Every day when I came home from work, I was hit by a fresh wave of pain that he wasn't there waiting for me, and it felt as though there was nothing to look forward to anymore. It was a genuine bereavement. However, I was young and busy so I did get through, or at least functioned as well as I could, even though I still felt heartbroken. I knew it was something that would never leave me.

I do wonder whether my reaction was disproportionate, but the truth is that I had gone from a difficult upbringing to a turbulent relationship. Again, it's something I don't really want to go into – the only important thing in my mind from that time is that I had a need to love and be loved. Animals could fill that hole in my heart and my life in a way that no person ever could. Buster had given me so much unconditional affection and I had felt able to return it without judgement or criticism – would I ever be able to do that again?

Six months after Buster had died, I did feel ready to welcome another little cat into my heart, but it didn't mean that I had forgotten Buster in any way, shape or form. I was terrified. I wanted to love but what if the same thing happened to another cat? Managing to overcome my fear, I brought Gertie into my life in 1989. A gorgeous tabby bundle of fluff, she soon became very feisty and had such a distinctive character. Tabby cats often have that attitude, and I was glad that she had a totally different personality to Buster. Another thing that helped was that, thankfully, Gertie only ever went out into the back garden, never out of the front door, so my fears were eased slightly. She would sit on the grass, rolling onto her back in the sun, and it always seemed as if she wanted to stay as close to home as possible.

'You're such a good girl,' I would say to her, as she sunbathed. 'You stay at home forever, do you hear me? You stay safe and sound so Mummy never loses you.' I'd give her a big kiss on her nose and I swear she looked at me as if she was taking in every word, and thinking, *Why on earth would I leave here? I've got you at my beck and call!*

Sadly, around the time I got Gertie, Pymmes died – she was more than twenty years old. I saw Mum grieve in a way I fully recognised. That cat had been her world and I knew that she would never get over the loss of her, just as I would never forget Buster. I know that there were people telling Mum just the things they had told me – *you'll get over it* or *she had a good life*, but it doesn't matter what age they are or how good you have made their lives, you just feel that gaping hole where their love used to be.

I believe animals come to you rather than you going to them. When you are blessed with a dog, cat or any other creature in your world, it's them who made the choice to come into it, not you. Even if you go to a rescue centre, you'll be chosen, not the other way about. The timid puppy who finds enough bravery to walk over and lick your hand;

the older cat who has been sitting at the back of her cage for months but who finally gets up to purr as you stroke her head; they are telling you, *I'm for you and you're for me.* There's a purity to that relationship that you'll never get from another human.

I also truly believe that I was an abused animal in a previous life. My soul hurts when I think of animal pain, and the fact that the feeling is so intense makes me feel that I must have been one once, that I must have gone through that too. I feel more settled with animals than I ever do with humans and I have very few friends. When I wonder where all this has all come from, it leads me back to the belief that I have been here before, maybe many times, and I am now in this world at this time and in this form to make a difference to these precious creatures.

During that earlier time in my life, though, I'm not sure that I had thought all of that through so clearly, as there were so many other things happening. I used to sit in the garden with Gertie, telling her all of my worries as she lolled about. She was a key part of my tiny family, and then my family grew. In 1991, my son, Bradley, was born. It wasn't the easiest time of my life as my baby basically had no immune system. He was in and out of hospital constantly while he was still very young. All I wanted was my little boy, but he was often hooked up to a drip.

'I'll learn,' I told the medical staff. 'I might not be a doctor or a nurse, but I'll learn. Teach me how to look after him, teach me everything to do with his drips and injections and medication, and I'll take the best care of him in the world. Just please, please, let me take him home for a little bit.'

Thankfully, they did. Luckily, I've never been squeamish and I soon knew just how to deal with it all. Thanks to the wonderful help of the hospital staff, and with a bit of time and patience, to my relief Bradley got to the stage where he was a perfectly happy and healthy little boy, but those were dark days for me as a new mother.

My relationship was still very difficult, and would remain so until we separated when I was in my thirties, but my beloved cat and my gorgeous little boy were two beautiful rays of hope in the middle of it all. Gertie always sat at the end of Bradley's cot; the two of us already had such a strong bond, so she never felt left out when Bradley arrived and we were a tight-knit group of three from the beginning. As Bradley grew, he was so gentle with her and I think they both knew from the start that they had special places in my heart. Of course, everyone loves their baby – or they should – but it was as if Bradley acknowledged from a very early age that I would never have pushed Gertie aside just because I had a child. That was my little family. I was happy with one baby and Gertie had been spayed, which meant no little ones for her, which meant that we were both mummies to Bradley.

In 1993, when my son was two, we moved to a bigger house with a large garden. Gertie kept to her old routine of staying nearby, lazing on the grass whenever she could. I'd see her from the kitchen window as I made dinner or did the washing-up, and this was always a comfort to me during very difficult personal times.

By now, you're probably wondering why I'm telling you so much about cats when you were promised dogs! The truth is, it was cats who were around so much at the beginning, and it was cats who made me realise that I loved animals so much. There were no dogs in my life at that point – but they would come in time.

I don't know why, but all the stray cats in the neighbourhood used to turn up in my garden. Maybe Gertie had passed word to the others, or maybe they sensed I was a soft touch once I fed the first strays, but it wasn't long before there was a whole gang of them hanging around. I wouldn't just feed them, I'd take them to the vet and make beds for them in winter. The beds were made from boxes lined with blankets and tinfoil to retain the heat, and I'd line them all up like a little dormitory. Sometimes I'd even find foxes in there when it was really cold.

I remember one day doing the family shop and the trolley was piled high with cat food.

'Oooh, you must have a few!' laughed the woman on the checkout.

I could feel myself flushing, knowing that, technically, I only had Gertie, but I couldn't admit to that given that I looked like I was shopping for about twenty of them!

'You know how it is!' I smiled. 'Cats can be fussy so best make sure I'm covered!'

I certainly was – I was covered for every cat in the neighbourhood, and that was just the start of it!

TWO

Crazy Cat Lady

Those cats came from far and wide, which was completely in line with my belief that animals find you, not the other way round. It wasn't long before I was known in our neighbourhood at the Crazy Cat Lady. Everyone in the area had heard of me, and it seemed like there was always someone else who had also heard of a cat or kitten who needed help. First of all, there was Kit Kat, who came to me in a roundabout way – someone knew someone who had spoken to someone else who had heard that a woman somewhere was getting rid of a cat and it would just be dumped.

At least, that's how the stories always sounded – they were often vague, but I could never turn away from helping an animal in need. Kit Kat was a gorgeous black and white boy, still young and so affectionate. He loved belly tickles and became a soppy lump when I sat for ages making a fuss of him. I think that stray cats are so prevalent because many of them are unneutered, so the litters multiply, and there are lots of feral cats around too. On top of that, cats have their own minds, and can often just take off, finding a new house, or they combine a few 'owners' to get what they want at different times. It certainly seemed as if there was a never-ending supply of cats in need out there!

After Kit Kat, there was Scooby. I was doing a car boot sale one weekend and got talking to a woman who worked at a cat rescue centre.

'We've got this lovely little lady there,' she said, 'but she's obviously the runt of the litter as she's so tiny, and no one will even look at her. I don't know if we'll ever find her a home.'

She'd barely finished her sentence before I said, 'I'll have her!' I couldn't bear the thought of some poor little fur baby being ignored for the rest of her life, when she could come and stay with my gang. I actually felt a physical pain when I thought of any animal going without love, not having a home and someone to snuggle up – if I could help, I would.

I was in full swing as the Crazy Cat Lady, and I would do whatever I could to help. However, I obviously couldn't take them all in, so I would take those most in need to the vet or leave out food for feral cats, anything that might make a difference. I never knew when there would be a knock on my door.

One day, a kid turned up with a cardboard box.

'You Michelle?' he asked, abruptly.

I looked suspiciously at the box, pretty sure there would be another kitty in there.

'Here,' he said, holding it out to me. 'Found this in the alley. I was told you would deal with it.'

Off he ran, leaving me with the most stunning tortoise-shell. 'Well, look at you!' I said to her. 'Are you coming to live with me now? I bet you are – you've come home, haven't you? Something has brought us together and this is where you'll be staying now.' She looked at me as if this was something she was perfectly aware of, and her eyes seemed to be asking me why had it taken me so long to find her!

I named her Lolly. What a cat she was! Completely independent, she never showed an ounce of affection unless she was in bed with me at night. At all other times, she'd sleep in a clean litter tray! Everything was on her terms, even if it was something that made her uncomfortable – like the litter tray! It was as if she was thinking, *Well, I know you want me to do that thing, so I will do the other thing . . . and you'll just have to accept it because I am queen of all I survey and you are there to jump to my every request!* She was spot-on, as was every cat I knew. It was as if they wrote their own contracts but didn't wait for you to sign them!

In the summer of 1999, I had another addition to the family – my daughter, Eloise. Gertie was still my little darling, and was always hanging around the kids, always looking out for them, and I just felt such a connection to her. I now had a house of children and cats, welcome distractions from the struggles I was going through in my relationship. I didn't really go out, unless it was to work, so any socialising was done at home. I'm not really someone who has lots of friends, or who needs huge gatherings – I'm happier with animals – but, not long after I'd had Eloise, guests did come round to ours for a bit of a get-together in the garden one day. It was a gloriously warm afternoon and the cats – including Gertie – all trotted about as people chatted and ate their al fresco lunch. Eloise was just a newborn and it was actually a really nice day: she was getting lots of attention, and her big brother was playing quite happily – it all gave the appearance of a very normal, perfectly happy family life, even though I knew that it could always change in the blink of an eye.

'I'm just popping out to the car for something,' said my friend Angela, handing the baby back to me. 'Won't be a moment.'

I walked around, bouncing Eloise on my hip and chatting to a few other people when, within seconds, Angela came running back into the garden.

'Oh my God, there's a cat been run over out there!' she screamed. 'The poor thing – it's just awful!'

My heart sank. I knew where all of mine were, but some poor soul was going to have their heart broken that day and I could feel that pain instantly in my chest. This would be the most awful day for someone, and I had flashbacks of losing my own fur babies.

'What does it look like, Angela?' I asked, knowing all the cats in the neighbourhood. 'I'll go tell the owners and they can come and collect the poor soul.'

'Tabby – definitely tabby,' she told me, tears in her eyes. 'I don't know what else, it was hard to tell – it was a tabby, that's all I took in.'

All of a sudden, a thought flitted across my mind and cold washed over me.

Gertie. Where was Gertie?

I hadn't seen her for a while, I realised. I'd thought she was just lying in the sun, and she never went out the front, but actually, she hadn't been around for about half an hour or so.

Dear God, no. Not my Gertie!

But it was. It was Gertie. Another friend who knew her went out to check and when he came back, I could just tell from the look on his face.

'I'm so sorry, Michelle – it's her.'

I fell to my knees sobbing. She'd been in my life for ten years and she'd never left the house or garden. Now, she was gone. How could life change in an instant, how could devastation be so immediate?

'Don't look – just stay out here and we'll take care of her,' said Angela. As the one who had first found Gertie, she was still shaking, but I knew – as did everyone else – that I was in no fit state to go out there and see that awful sight. Angela went back indoors, up to my bedroom, and came down with a beautiful blue vanity case of mine that she'd emptied out. She and another friend went to the front of the house and tenderly placed my gorgeous girl in the padded satin case.

'We'll take her to the vet,' said Angela, holding me in her arms as I shook with grief.

'No!' I said, instantly. 'I've had her ten years – I need her with me for longer. Don't take her away from me, please don't. Please let me keep her beside me.'

Everyone pulled together that afternoon. They dug a hole in the garden in the most beautiful sunny spot and that's where my Gertie was laid to rest. We laid flowers there and I made plans to plant a beautiful rose bush that would bloom in her honour. I'm not sure how I got through the rest of that day, or the ones that followed. Naturally, most people left once they had comforted me and passed on their condolences, but there was the same feeling with some that they couldn't quite work out why I was in such a state. Angela stayed and helped with the kids, and I kept playing over and over in my mind what it must have been like for Gertie. I don't think she had been lying there for long, as I would have missed her, but my heart broke for the fact that she had been alone.

I never found out who had run her over and, to be honest, that's probably for the best as I wouldn't have been able to control myself. They had taken her from me and the ten years we'd had wasn't enough by any means.

It was a real bereavement, a genuine loss. Was it worse than Buster? I don't think you can compare one pet with another. You love them all and you grieve for them all. Our time together is limited from the moment they come into our lives, and they'll always cross over Rainbow Bridge too soon. However, I did worry constantly about roads and cats, and there was a part of me that wondered if I would lose them all that way. I wished I could just keep them safe by me forever, but, as I have said before, cats are their own bosses and you just can't make them abide by your rules, even if those rules are to make them safe.

I still helped out with local cats whenever I could but didn't take a new one into my home until Eloise was a toddler. The kids were taking up a lot of my time and I was juggling life's demands, like all women do, but it was clear by then that Eloise was a magnet for animals, just like her mum. She loved her guinea pigs and hamsters, and all of our cats hung around her whenever they got a chance. She was a lovely little girl, so gentle with all of them, and I felt that she too would be a caring friend for all living creatures as she grew up.

I believe that once you open your heart to animals, they are drawn to you, and it becomes so hard to say 'no' that you just don't bother to anymore. Saying 'yes' brings so much more love into your life. The next one to move into Chez Michelle was Pickle, and that was the start of our household getting bigger and bigger.

The phone rang one morning out of the blue, and I was surprised to hear the vet on the other end of the line. All my cats were up to date with their vaccinations, so I couldn't think why she was calling.

'We've got a lovely little black and white cat here,' she explained.

Here we go, I thought.

'What's the story?' I asked, not sure whether to be delighted at the thought of another addition to the family or wonder how I was going to stop people seeing me as a soft touch! However, I was happy to open up my home when I could, and did feel there was still space, so asking after this little one could do no harm, I told myself.

'It's appalling,' she told me. 'The poor soul only has alopecia, but the owners don't want to pay for treatment, so have decided to give her up.'

Alopecia! The cat had bald patches, hair falling out. I understood that vet treatments could be expensive, and I know that financial hardship can lead to people being forced to give up their animals, but it sounded to me as though the owners were going to get rid of this poor cat because they saw her as something to just cast aside. It's stories like this that infuriate me because I always suspect that the people who have dumped their pet see them as disposable. If I had a little cat or dog in that position, I'd scrimp and save, I'd be the one to go without, just to make sure they got the treatment they needed. These are living souls; they feel and they understand. I will never be able to work out how some people can just distance themselves from those facts. Sadly, I was to come across it a lot more as the years went on.

'I'll be there as soon as I can,' I sighed.

'You're a saint, Michelle,' the vet replied.

'A daft one,' I laughed. Off I went to Chingford with a cat basket, and back I came with Pickle. That cat took to Eloise instantly, idolising her from the outset and moaning non-stop if she wasn't there. With the right treatment and a lot of love, Pickle was soon on the mend, and I was so thankful that the vet had called me when this poor cat had been unceremoniously dumped through absolutely no fault of her own.

When I wasn't being brought cats, I was finding them. I was walking home from the shops one day and passed a small piece of open land, close to a junkyard. I could hear a meow and I kept trying to work out where it was coming from, but the pouring rain was so loud that it was hard to hear anything. Finally, my ears attuned and I followed the noise – only to find a scraggy little cat and six tiny kittens. The yard was less than five minutes from my house, so I ran home and got a carrier.

When I got back to the junkyard, my heart was pounding and I was drenched. I'd popped a fleecy blanket into the carrier to make it warm and cosy for this little family and I desperately wanted to get them in there and to safety.

'Oh my goodness, look at the size of you,' I whispered gently to them as I carefully put them inside the basket. Their little noises were so tiny, so pathetic, and I dreaded to think what would have happened to them had I not heard them in that awful weather. 'You are the most gorgeous little creatures, aren't you? Now, let's get you and your mummy checked over.'

I took them to a local cat charity as that was closer than the vet, where I was told that they were only a day old. They also told me that they didn't have the capacity to take them in as they were full, so I should just return them to the yard where I'd found them!

'I can't just leave them! They'll never survive out there. What the hell do I do with seven cats?' I asked – but I knew the answer even as the words came out of my mouth. I took them home. They were the most delightful little things and I was so privileged to see them from such an early stage. I knew I couldn't keep them all – seven! – but I would cross that bridge when I came to it.

Then there was Freddie.

'Guess what I've found?' my friend Hayley said to me one day.

'I'm going to really go wild here,' I laughed. 'Any chance it's a cat?'

'Four actually,' she admitted, 'four little kittens in someone's back garden and no mum to be seen.'

'Oh Hayley,' I wailed. 'Four little lost souls! I'd love to, but you know how many I have.'

'But there's good news!' she told me. 'I've found homes for three of them, but not the runt. He's gorgeous, Michelle, you'll love him.'

I had to hand it to Hayley, that was a good approach – to make me think she needed me to take four, when it was 'only' another one, was a skilled manoeuvre! Of course, I couldn't say no.

'Go on then,' I said, only confirming what I bet Hayley knew all along, 'I'll have him.'

Freddie turned into this huge fluffy black cat with white splodges, and, as I'm writing this, he's rolling about in the sunshine, which is streaming through the window, a bit battered and scruffy-looking now that he's twelve, but he is truly one of the best cats I've ever known. He can become a bit crazy, but I have a special whistle that I blow when I need him to calm down. It's like magic and makes me feel like an animal whisperer! He's always adored me and still scrambles up on to the end of the bath when I'm having a soak. But when I first got him, I ran into a stumbling block, as the Mummy cat that I'd rescued from the yard hated him on sight.

Once I'd brought her and her babies back with me, I set about finding homes for them, but I wanted to keep her as she'd had such a hard time. I named her Minnae and it was as if she decided that I was her mother from the moment I took her into my life. I managed to find homes for all of the kittens apart from the tiniest – Betty – who I was still bottle-feeding as Minnae couldn't manage them all. Both Minnae and Freddie wanted to be glued to me 24/7, but Minnae was more assertive, and she'd hiss at Freddie if he was ever in my arms, although she wasn't like that with any of the others. I had seven cats and two toddlers at this point, and it seemed I'd always be the Crazy Cat Lady. This would just be my life. I'd rescue cats and have them brought to me by everyone in the neighbourhood. I'd answer the door to children with scraggy moggies in their arms and I'd be the first port of call for any abandoned animals at the vets, any time I took one of mine in for a check-up or treatment. Something bigger than me had decided this was to be my life, and I was fine with that.

I had no idea what was waiting around the corner for me.

THREE

Just Where I Needed to Be

Time passed – children, cats, life, and I also set up a few businesses of my own. I had a sunbed shop, a baby shoes business and quite a few others. It was exhausting juggling family life with work, though, and I sometimes felt as if I spent all day driving from one place to another, with no time for myself, and small children to bring up into the bargain. I never really felt satisfied though, so I would start up yet another sideline, probably in the hope that something would stick, that I'd find something that would feel like 'me'.

So, in 2010, a friend and I set up a group called 'Cause for Paws'. We both loved animals and were horrified at there being so many without homes. Far too many of them were being slung out when people got fed up with them, as if they were rubbish to be thrown onto the streets.

'This is just awful,' I said to my friend Debbie. 'It breaks my heart to see this happening – I need to do something. Are you in?'

'I'm not sure what you're thinking of,' she replied, 'but, yeah, let's see what we can do!'

It had to be quite an informal setting, as doing something as major as setting up a charity is very complicated and time-consuming, but these cats and dogs didn't need anything fancy. Debbie and I did as much fundraising as we could find time for and found foster homes as well as forever homes wherever possible. Everything was done solely through our Facebook page, but before long we were being inundated with messages, either from people wanting to get rid of a dog or those who knew of one who had been dumped. It turned out that, for the most part, we were dealing with Staffies – there seemed to be a complete overflow of them. I didn't really know that much about the breed until I started dealing with them on a constant basis, and I soon found out that many people were automatically prejudiced against them. Although they had originally been bred as fighting dogs, that was hundreds of years ago, and I've always found them to be sweet, placid souls. Sadly, too often they were seen as a symbol of the owner being 'hard', rather than the gentle, loyal dogs they are when treated well. They bond so well with their owners, even when those owners don't deserve them. I don't believe there is any such thing as a 'bad' dog, but I was seeing plenty of humans who didn't deserve to have such loving creatures in their lives.

The more I learned about Staffies, the more I loved them. They are such affectionate dogs, with a tendency to stick like glue to their owner, and a real need for cuddles. However, the influx of them – and other dogs and cats – was absolutely overwhelming. There was an intensity that was hard for our informal little group to cope with, and we had to wind it down. Neither Debbie or I had been prepared for what we were going to be faced with – and given that I could never say 'no' to a dog in need, it was becoming a real struggle.

In 2012, I began a job working at a detection centre. A friend was working there, on the training side, and needed someone to help out. I took up the offer and became responsible for all of the administrative work and staff. This was a place where handlers and dogs were employed to search for explosives in grounds such as football stadiums, or buildings or entrance points. The handlers and dogs were highly trained and had become a vital part of the ongoing process to be vigilant against any individual or group who might want to cause harm, particularly at a large event. I wasn't one of the handlers, but I was very much involved in the company, making sure that citizens and military personnel were as safe as possible. This job was yet another contact with the canine rather than feline world, and I realised I had taken to it as if it was the most natural thing in the world, which, for me, it turned out to be!

In my first year, I worked at the London Olympics, which was a huge undertaking with lots of explosive search dogs – or explo-dogs as they are known. I was in the office in the athletes' village, which was a fabulous experience. The dogs, the atmosphere, the people; it was so uplifting and an honour to be involved in such an event. I don't think anyone had anticipated just how much it would mean to the country; I also doubt they had much idea of what was going on behind the scenes. Our dogs were busy from the start, having to get all of the scent-work done from the opening ceremony onwards. They were all Springer Spaniels, keen dogs with a high drive. There was one black-and-white little character called Bailey, who was drawn to me immediately, and he would always come and sit with me when I was off duty. I fell in love with him instantly. I'd sneak in treats for him and he'd look at me with his big brown eyes as if I was the centre of his world!

'Oh Bailey,' I would say to him quietly, 'you are just a little darling – I'm going to miss you so much when we both move on from here.'

He'd gaze at me as if we were meant to be together, but I was no explo-dog handler, and I knew our time together was limited. After the Olympics, I was deployed to the training centre. The handlers were all ex-services, and most of the dogs were released to them by the company after the Olympics were over. I was delighted when I found out that Bailey was going to be there, and when I saw him again, I dropped to my knees and gave him such a big cuddle.

'Will you still be bringing him here every day?' I asked his handler, hopefully.

'I'm not taking him,' he replied. 'He's seven now, it's time for Bailey to retire. He's too old for this type of work. No, he'll be looking for somewhere else – I've got no idea where, to be honest.'

'I'll take him!' I shouted, immediately.

The handler looked at me in shock. I think I had maybe come across as just a little bit too enthusiastic!

'Nothing to do with me,' he said, shrugging. 'There must be procedures you go through.'

I rushed back to the office and asked my manager how I could get one of the dogs if he was retiring. I honestly didn't know if they would take me seriously, but he told me the way to go about it and I went home with Bailey that very night! He was going to have to live with seven cats – Kit Kat, Scooby, Minnae, Betty, Lolly, Freddie and Pickle – and I had no idea how that would work. What if they hated him? I needn't have worried – none of them were bothered in the slightest. There was no hissing, no chasing, they just all accepted him without question. Bailey walked in and settled immediately, as if he was meant to be there – which I felt he was.

I always felt that Bailey was born to be a therapy dog. He was such a gentle, kind soul that I could picture him sitting beside people in hospital, giving them comfort, or perhaps going into care homes and cheering up the elderly. If I'd had the time to do it, I would definitely have taken that path with him as I think assistance and therapy dogs are just incredible. I was absolutely delighted to have him in my life but, with so many animals now, I knew it was only a matter of time before there would be sadness again. Nevertheless, it was still a shock when Scooby and Kit Kat passed within only three months of each other.

The day after Scooby died, my son Bradley came home with a tiny silver tabby for me. I must admit, I was cross. He was only a young lad, but my grief over Scooby was consuming me, and I just wasn't ready to consider bringing another cat into my life.

'You can't just replace one animal with another – it doesn't work that way,' I told him.

His tearful face got to me though, and I just accepted that, as a mum, sometimes you have to let your emotions take second place and go with what your child desperately wants.

Timmy really was an adorable little cat and it became evident from that very first day that he was there for a reason. His relationship with Bailey was beautiful from the outset and they were inseparable, with the most amazing bond and friendship. They snuggled up, just those two together, all the time. Timmy would nestle under Bailey, curling up against his tummy to sleep. I didn't get a look in! It was such a lovely friendship but, at nine months old, Timmy started becoming unwell. After many visits to the vet, it was determined that he had a rare type of kidney tumour and there was nothing they could do. I wanted a transplant for him but that wasn't an option. He stayed at the vet's for a week while they ran all sorts of tests and then, when he finally got home, it was as if Bailey knew. I had been keeping him up to date after every phone call, and he always sat there with his head cocked to the side as if he understood it all. When Timmy came home, I genuinely felt as though Bailey knew what was happening.

I slept downstairs with Timmy in my arms and Bailey lying as close to us as he could manage. During the day, Bailey would be the one who cared for and nurtured him. That dog was an angel. One of those nights, I had finally fallen asleep, exhausted with worry, with little Timmy fitfully napping in my arms, when Bailey started nudging me.

'Oh Bailey,' I said groggily, my eyelids too heavy to lift. 'Mummy's exhausted – just wait until morning, then I can play with you.'

I scratched his ear a bit, but he wouldn't stop whining and his pawing was becoming increasingly frantic. I opened my eyes to see Timmy unresponsive in my arms. I rushed him to the vet, promising Bailey I would do all I could for his little friend as I closed the door behind me, but there was nothing they could do. Timmy had gone. It was so sad and Bailey just didn't know what to do. He was completely bereft and I felt as if we were grieving together. He had loved that little cat as much I had, and we spent many hours together, missing him terribly.

Not long after Timmy passed, there was another addition to our gang – it did seem as if I was well and truly the Crazy Cat *and* Dog Lady now! I had a friend who had purchased a Maltese terrier puppy from abroad. As soon as it arrived, it seemed obvious to me that it was from a puppy farm. The poor little girl was underweight, poorly and very scared. By the time she was seven months old, my friend wasn't able to provide the dog with what she needed, and said she'd have to get rid of Milly.

'I'll have her,' I said, without hesitation. Again, I feel that all this happened for a reason. Within two days, Milly had to be taken to see the vet as it turned out that she had acute pancreatitis. I would always move heaven and earth to save any animal, money no object, so I was just glad that she was with me rather than a family who couldn't provide her with all that she needed.

I went to see Milly every single day while she was being looked after at the practice.

'You'll pull through,' I always told her. 'You were meant to be here, with me, and you are strong – you haven't survived this long for it to end now.' She did pull through at that point, but her health kept dropping and the pancreatitis would return frequently. There were months of care and medication needed, and, when Milly was at her worst, she would be on a drip. I begged the vet to let me take her home even though she was hooked up to it, but they were against it, telling me that it was a huge responsibility and a 24/7 commitment. I was used to this because of my experiences when Bradley was little. Back then, he had been allowed home with a drip on more than one occasion and I'd learned to deal with it, so Milly's predicament was one I felt confident that I could handle. It was tough but she got on OK. She was full of fire and feisty – a bit like me! – a survivor and fiercely loyal for such a tiny scrap of a thing. She did perk up, although she was never 100 per cent fighting fit, but she slotted in so well. It's as if all my animals know that they need love and that they will get unlimited amounts from me. They all got on well with each other too. Milly was the baby, even smaller than most of the cats, but she had the heart of a lion.

In 2013, I left the detection dog company and set up an online pet toy business. I was back to spending an awful lot of my time driving between suppliers and outlets, distributors and shops. I used to drive through Crouch End almost every day. There were traffic lights outside a Waitrose that never seemed to be in my favour, and I'd sit there, mentally running through the list of a million things I had to do that day. Out of the corner of my eye, I often saw the same man sitting in the doorway of the shop. No matter the weather, he'd be there with his Staffie beside him. I was completely naïve and genuinely couldn't work out why someone would just sit there, not moving, rain or shine, with a dog who seemed so placid that it never moved either.

It was the dog that I connected with, and any time I sat at the traffic lights, I would look over, checking he was still there – for some reason I assumed it was a boy – and always felt a wave of relief when I saw him sitting there quietly, curled up close to his owner. *That's no life for a dog though*, I would think to myself. He needs walks and treats, he needs a better life than just sitting there, day in, day out. I still hadn't comprehended why the man was always there with his dog.

It was a few weeks until Christmas, and I decided I needed to do something for this creature. I got one of those old mushroom boxes with silver handles and filled it with toys and treats for the dog. Even if he was just there with nothing to do, I reasoned he could at least munch on some tasty things or gnaw on a toy to keep him occupied. I didn't have the courage to do anything though, and it took me a week to gear myself up enough to pull in, park, and go over to them. I was intrigued to know why they were both always just sitting there, but I also felt really nervous.

I finally walked over, the Christmas box for the dog in my bag, and stopped in front of them.

'Hello,' I said. 'I see you here every day, don't I?' The man looked up at me but all I could see was that the dog's tail had started to wag. 'I hope I'm not intruding, but do you mind if I ask you why?'

'Why what?' the man asked, looking confused.

'Why are you here every day?' I repeated.

He looked at me as if I had two heads – which, in retrospect, he had every right to do as I was being completely ridiculous and utterly naïve.

'Why am I here every day?' he parroted back to me as I nodded. 'I'm here every day because I'm homeless, that's why.'

'You don't have a home? You don't have a home at all?' I asked, shocked. (I'm cringing at the very memory, even as I write this!)

'No,' he said, patiently. 'I sleep outside. Just me and my dog.'

I couldn't grasp it. I couldn't grasp that someone would spend their day in a shop doorway, waiting for a few coins or a sandwich, with their dog beside them and not have some-where to go to at night. Winter was fast approaching and the temperature was already dropping at night, combined with it raining most of the time – and that beautiful dog had no fire to curl up in front of, no basket to snooze in until morning. Then, even when morning did come, it was still the same old doorway.

'I'm Michelle – what's your name?' I asked.

'Kenneth – and this is Prince.' At the mere mention of his dog's name, Kenneth finally smiled, and it transformed his whole face.

'I've got something for Prince!' I told him. 'A Christmas present!' I handed over the box to Kenneth as Prince came over to it, sniffing and giving one of those smiles that I would come to think of as a Staffie trademark. Kenneth's face had lit up as soon as I said I had something for his dog and, now he seemed completely overwhelmed.

'Look at this, boy!' he said as Prince was getting more and more excited, no doubt smelling some of the treats inside. 'Look at the tinsel! Look at all these things for you!'

I was crouched down beside them both and felt so happy, choked up really, that they both had this moment of pleasure in their day. I also couldn't help but notice the way that people were just walking by, heads down, not really registering Kenneth and Prince. Of course, that could have been because I was there, but when I thought of how little I understood, it was only natural that many of them would have felt the same way too, and probably didn't even notice him as they did their shopping. I felt so guilty that I had only given them a box, and that I didn't even have anything for Kenneth. I left them, feeling just as overwhelmed as they seemed to be, but I'd only gone a few steps when he shouted out, 'Michelle, Michelle!'

I turned around and Kenneth was smiling as if he'd won the lottery. 'This was our lucky day, wasn't it? We were just where we needed to be today!'

I smiled and kept glancing back over my shoulder as I walked back to the car. Maybe this was just where I had needed to be that day as well.

FOUR

A Hidden World

I went back to see Kenneth and Prince after about a week, once Christmas had passed. I was still naïve and had so many questions for him:

Why wasn't the council helping?

Why wasn't his family helping?

Why weren't friends helping?

How did he wash and bathe?

How did he stay warm?

What happened if he was ill?

What happened if Prince was ill?

Did he always get enough to eat?

Did the shop mind him being there?

Were people mean or cruel or dismissive?

Did some people help?

What kind of help was best?

I must have driven him mad, but he was so patient with me. I'd never ask those questions now – not because I know all of the answers, the practical side of things, but because it isn't my place to intrude. If someone wants to tell me their story, they will. I became switched on to it. Homelessness was on my radar now and I'd see more and more people living on the streets wherever I went – and so many dogs. It broke my heart and it felt as if I was following a trail of them through Central London. Everywhere I looked, there were multitudes of people in sleeping bags with dogs, their worldly possessions by their sides.

The pet toy business was taking me more and more into the heart of London, so maybe that's why I was so aware of it, but I did feel as if I just hadn't opened my eyes before I'd met Kenneth and Prince. We can all be so locked in our own little worlds, worrying about things that in reality are so insignificant when you think of what these people are going through. I'd be driving, stressed, thinking of when I'd get the chance to pop into the supermarket later and grab something for dinner, while people on the streets didn't know where their next meal was coming from. I'd be stressing about how there weren't enough hours in the day, while homeless people just saw one day blend into another, with no focus, nothing to look forward to. I'd had a real wake-up call and knew from that point on that there were so many Kenneths and Princes out there that maybe, just maybe, I could do something to help.

In my mind, there was a slight warning from Cause for Paws, the previous dog aid group I had tried to run on

Facebook. It had become overwhelming very quickly and I'd learned that I did have a problem in saying 'no' when it came to animals, but maybe I could learn from those experiences, and perhaps if I had a more specific goal in mind, it would be easier to not be overwhelmed by the sheer scale of the problem.

I started parking up whenever I had the chance, just watching how many people there were sleeping rough, before plucking up the courage to walk over and start talking to them. It wasn't that I was afraid, and I've never been exactly shy, but I just didn't want to impose. I didn't want to be one of those people who just parachutes in and then does nothing. Once I'd introduced myself and chatted a bit, I asked the one question that I hoped would matter.

'What do you need?'

Socks, came the answer, time and time again. It was always socks.

I was puzzled at first – I had assumed that perhaps they'd want blankets, or something more luxurious than a simple pair of socks. But the more time I spent talking to people, the more I came to gain some understanding about what it really meant to be living on the streets. Many of these people would spend hours walking or sitting on the cold, wet streets of London, more often than not in shoes that had seen better days. Having an extra, dry, clean pair of socks could make a real difference.

With a new mission in mind, I set about getting as many socks as I possibly could. I set up a Twitter account and a Facebook page for people to donate pairs of socks in all different sizes, and was thrilled when they started flooding in. Then I had a brainwave. If people's feet were cold in this weather, wouldn't their dogs' feet be cold too? So I asked for baby socks as well. I was inundated. Taking those socks to people and their dogs really broke down the barriers and helped me learn more about the challenges they faced.

It was a pleasure getting to know these people, most of whom were friendly and appreciative, and it felt good to know that I was doing something that could make a difference to their lives and help make their day-to-day experience just a little more comfortable.

It had taken off quickly and I felt a purpose from that first pair of socks onwards. I had an affinity with those people and their dogs from the start. I soon realised that street people are special people. They very rarely ask for anything and they're used to being invisible. But the dogs – the dogs were what hit me so hard. These were wonderful creatures, so caring and loving, so amazing in the way they approached everything. Street dogs are unwaveringly loyal to their owners. They are each other's entire worlds, and the bond between them is unbreakable. Imagine having very little in your life apart from a trusted companion. Imagine both of you trying to sleep in the freezing cold. Imagine having to choose between the safety of a bed for the night or staying with your dog – because that, I soon realised, was what happened. It's all very well for do-gooders to say that there are hostels available, that no one *really* needs to sleep on the streets, but when they have to decide between a roof over their head and leaving their dog, what kind of choice do they really have? Where would the dog go? Abandoned, to wait for their owner to come back the next day with absolutely no understanding of what was happening? Can you imagine the heartbreak of that for an animal who has only ever shown unwavering devotion and loyalty? For a lot of rough sleepers, their dog is their lifeline – their one remaining connection to another living creature that truly loves and cares for them.

The bond is unique and neither one would choose themselves over the other. Rain, sun, sleet, snow, hailstones, gales – they have to suffer it all, no matter how extreme, and they would rather suffer it together than ever dream of separating. There must have been about a quarter of street-homeless who had dogs at that point – it wasn't as common as it is now, but I loved meeting a person who had a dog, as animals were still my main passion – I'd just found another cause to add to the list.

I became obsessed. I started to meet homeless people every day, sock donations grew into donations of clothes, then sleeping bags, dog food, and of course, pet toys and treats for these precious creatures.

Speaking to these individuals about how they had found themselves in these positions opened my eyes to the difficulties faced by so many people, and it really brought home to me just how lives could change in a flash. One such person was a man named John, an ex-army medic who wandered through London every day with a sign saying he was desperate for work – he just wanted to be off the streets. But without a permanent address, no access to some of the basic necessities we all take for granted, he was trapped in a vicious cycle.

I got John a little mobile phone to keep in touch with him, and to help him on the first step to making a new life for himself. On Boxing Day, the phone rang, and I was surprised to hear John's voice on the other end of the line. He sounded desperate, and my heart was in my throat when he said, 'I can't do this any longer, Michelle.'

I managed to calm him down enough to tell me where he was, and begged him to wait for me there. I rushed from the house and drove to him, put him in a Travelodge (he didn't have a dog), and got him safe again. Sometimes we all just need a little kindness, and it really felt like a privilege to be able to help in any way I could.

I was focused on helping these people as much as possible, especially at that time of year, and I knew that something more needed to be done to support John and get him to a better place. I put a call-out on social media asking for donations to keep John safe, as there were no services open at that time of year to help him. As he didn't have a dog, I was able to get him into accommodation. I helped him sort his benefits and all the things needed to get him on the right path, organising interviews for longer-term private rented accommodation, where he still lives today and, eventually, work and a permanent job. I was determined that John never felt as low again as he had that day. It was all made worth it when he was finally offered a job, which was what he had needed all along. It just takes one person to believe in you to transform a life, and that was one of the main things John taught me. He's still working there to this day, and he is happy and contented, able to live like any other person.

Of course, I didn't know back then that there could be such huge successes as John because there seemed to be an overwhelming number of horrendous stories everywhere. I met women who had suffered terrible traumas in their lives; women who had been abused, who had fallen into bad relationships, been introduced to drink or drugs, and who were now being sold for sex and kept in slavery to feed their addictions, only to be kicked out onto the streets once they had served their purpose. It broke my heart that these women had no one else to turn to, that they had been let down at every turn by the very people who were supposed to care for them.

There were homeless men who had never told their families what position they were in because they were too ashamed and embarrassed. I even met one man whose children thought that he worked abroad and would come back one day. There were people who pretended that they had moved to a different part of the country when actually they were living very close to their estranged families, who would never have recognised them after years on the streets. All of these people needed a genuine friendship, someone to listen and support them, and I was more than happy to provide that. I'd listen as long as they wanted to talk or sit there in silence if that was what they needed. I never judged anyone for their choices and I never imposed on their lives. I just wanted to help in some small way.

For the five years that I ran my own outreach programme, what these people didn't know was that they were giving me so much too. Whilst it might have appeared that I was simply helping them, the sense of purpose and pleasure I felt at being able to help or make some small difference was amazing. I'd go home and I'd want to get back out immediately. I knew that there was another world, hidden to a lot of people – or deliberately ignored by them – that I had been given access to and all I wanted to do was be there, help where I could, and make sure they and their dogs were okay.

Most of these people had mental health issues – in fact, I struggle to think of anyone who didn't, and I'd be lying if I painted them all as saints. There were high levels of drug and alcohol addiction, but despite all of these challenges, there was a lot of laughter and unquestioning acceptance of me. I'd never really had that before. It was a bit surreal and I really enjoyed being with them. They quickly made me realise what was real and genuine in life. They spoke the hard truth, and they were raw friendships. I was never lied to. Coming from my background, where I'd had a very difficult childhood then gone straight into troubled relationship, this was another way of being. I'd felt invisible with what I'd gone through in life and yet I now felt recognised by the very community the rest of the world ignored. They gave me as much as I gave them. I was somebody to them and they had no idea what that meant to me.

I was giving them consistency. It was personal, not just someone sitting behind a desk and clocking out when their shift was over. Each person I got to know was an individual with their own history, their own pain, their own hopes and dreams for the future. I started going out every night, so the street homeless saw me regularly and I knew them as people, not as cases or file numbers. This wasn't my job; it was my calling.

From that moment just before Christmas when I first spoke to Kenneth and Prince, to the spring of 2013, I learned more than I could ever have imagined. Yes, it was an intense experience, but it was something that could never have been found in books or on courses. This was real life with real people. Their day-to-day world was something that wasn't an experiment, or an oddity to poke about at. They weren't in a zoo, or some sort of museum piece, they were human beings who, for some reason or another, had found themselves in a position they couldn't get themselves out of. The more I found out about the so-called support they had, the less I wondered about why there were still so many people living on the streets. There was so little in the way of a safety net to protect a person from homelessness, and it seemed to me that, unless you were able to jump through every hoop and fit into every neat category, it was incredibly difficult to get any help at all. I felt frustrated at the way that most services operated, with no flexibility or understanding of the reality of these people's lives, lives that had gone off the rails at some point.

I'd drive into Central London from home and park at Westminster or by Charing Cross Police Station. It would already be cold and dark, and even on the weekend mornings when I could get there early, there were days that never really got light, and when the temperature never got above freezing. I had my thick socks, a padded coat, warm trousers and a jumper, layer upon layer, gloves, a scarf, a hat – and was often still cold. No matter where I parked, no matter where I walked, there were homeless people, and none of them had the benefit of what I was wearing. I soon realised that one of the main things I could do was ask everyone I knew for donations, whether they were bought or were from having a clearout. Whenever I had enough, I would take out a suitcase or holdall and fill it with hats, scarves, socks, thermals, handwarmers, trainers, anything I had been given that was in good condition. From that point, I made a promise to myself that I would never give these people rubbish or hand-me-downs that were only really fit for going in the bin. They deserved decent things and they certainly deserved not to be treated as human waste bins. I was furious if anyone ever gave me overworn tatty clothes or socks with holes in them that couldn't be mended, things that really just needed to be thrown out, because what message did that send to the recipient? You could get a big pack of socks for a fiver, a padded coat for twenty quid in one of the big discount stores, and I'd much rather spend my own money on new things like that for people than give them something that was barely fit for purpose anymore. Some of my friends were very kind though, and I ended up with quite a lot of supplies that winter, and the ones which followed.

I was learning every day. One thing that did surprise me was that a lot of the street homeless had families and friends. I couldn't imagine ever letting a loved one sleep on the streets, and I'd assumed that people with that sort of network could sofa-surf. It turned out that many didn't have that option. There was often huge embarrassment at the reality of their lives and they would have done anything to make sure that no one ever found out the dire straits they were in. As I've mentioned, some had children who believed their fathers were working abroad indefinitely, and many of them had relied on the hospitality of friends to begin with, but pretended that things were looking up and moved out when they felt they had outstayed their welcome. Nobody ever wanted to feel that they were a burden, and I respected them for their sense of pride and self-preservation, in spite of the terrible things they had endured.

For some people, the streets were the only option – for too many people, in my mind. There were few places that gave a real helping hand, long term, to those with problems such as relationship breakdowns, debt, gambling, addictions, family fights, rent arrears, and all the issues that came with broken lives. It was frightening to see how quickly a life could spiral out of control. All it could take was one small change to cause a person just like you or me to suddenly find themselves with no option but to sleep rough. A lot of the men, especially, felt that they couldn't turn to families and friends, as they hated to be questioned or judged; they didn't want anyone to think that they had failed at being a man.

I didn't question them or the decisions that had brought them to this point, I was just there to help in that moment. My first priority was to show them that I was there if they needed me, and that someone would help without judging. Everyone has a story, but it's up to them to tell it in their own time. I believed they should make their own decisions and choices. I'd just ask questions that related to how I could help, rather than demanding their life story before I acted like Lady Bountiful dishing out little bits of charity here and there. 'What can I do? What do you want?'

We all have our problems and hardships, whether you have a roof or not. Those of us with homes are just more fortunate, but the reality is that there's very little to separate 'us' from 'them'. Homeless people are often made to feel invisible – most people barely seem to notice them, or else perhaps they were too embarrassed to stop. As a result, those living on the streets feel so looked down upon by the world that they think there's nothing left, and no hope anymore.

Despite people's preconceptions about homeless people and substance abuse, they only ever asked me for practical stuff. I'd get them Pay-as-You-Go phones and give them my personal number that they only used in emergencies or if they hadn't seen me for a while and needed something.

It wasn't long before I was out on the streets of London every night from 2 p.m. until midnight. I was drawn to helping these people in an almost obsessive way that I could barely understand. I'd sit on the ground with coffee and cake and people-watch until someone decided they wanted to come up to me, perhaps because someone said I had helped, perhaps because they were just curious. In time, I was able to gain people's trust, and they learned that there was someone there who was giving their time without asking for anything back. That was the most important first step of all.

I walked those streets around Westminster until I knew them as well as my own house. I'd look at the Houses of

Parliament, at the Commons and the Lords, there to represent us, there for us, to protect and support us, and I would think, *You have no idea*. I'm not a particularly political person and I didn't think this in terms of one party or another – I just wished that the people in power, who made decisions, could truly see what was happening in the streets where they walked every day.

I never felt worried or threatened when I was out on the streets. I'd just start every conversation the same way.

'Hi, I'm Michelle. What's your name? What can I do to help? Can I get you a coffee?'

I was touched that people started looking out for me, worrying about me if I was straying too far, going to places they thought I shouldn't be. Soho was one of those places.

'You're not going there on your own,' they would tell me, but if I was insistent, if I'd heard of a person or an animal who really needed help, I had to go. To my surprise, they would make sure that two or three people went with me. We must have made a strange-looking gang to those who passed us, me with my make-up and manicure, sorted for any weather, and a couple of homeless people carrying their lives in a bag, all walking along, having a laugh.

Everything was a two-way street once we got to know each other, and they would always ask me about my day. In that respect, they were often better friends than those in my 'other' life who could sometimes be very dismissive of what I was doing with the street homeless, or who came to the whole subject with a lot of preconceived ideas based, to be perfectly honest, on ignorance.

I quickly learned that the people I helped, or met with a plan to help, never disclosed things straight away, and I think that was because they had been burned so often in the past, by people who had made promises to help them. Support groups, street help, case workers – all of them have their place when they help, and there are some that do terrific jobs, but they can also act as if they will change the world for an individual one moment, and then be very limited in what they could provide the next. I never overpromised, never said I could do more than I was able to. All I offered to start with was a coffee – and they knew that was something they'd get if nothing else. Once I had their trust, they started to answer the other question: 'What can I do for you, how can I help now?' There was so much. Clothes. Food. Medicine. Registering with a GP. Help to access washing facilities. Little things that we all take for granted, but which aren't even options for the hidden people.

Now that I knew they were there, now that I'd had my eyes opened, I promised myself I would never turn my back again.

FIVE

Finding Friends

The first thing most people ask someone homeless is, 'Why are you here?' They want to know what happened to them, they want to know whether they deserve help or whether that person can be blamed for their own situation. So most homeless people make up a little story, probably not the whole truth, although there may be a smattering of it in there, because they don't want to hang their lives out to dry for every stranger who needs their curiosity satisfied.

I wouldn't want to be endlessly questioned about my life every day, would you? These people are on show because of certain circumstances in their lives, but why should they be forced to look back at their own heartache constantly, all for the sake of a cheap sandwich or a pound thrown in a paper cup? It's a sad state of affairs when another human being has to try and work out what story you will accept before you help them. Some people like to believe in a kind of 'perfect victim', but there's no such thing. Everyone has their own story, everyone has found themselves in their current position for different reasons, but whatever those reasons are, there's nothing that could make me feel that one person is more worthy of help than another.

That's partly the reason why I don't bother asking people how they came to be in the position they're in now – what would be the benefit in them spinning me a tale, and what would it change?

Once I had been doing my own outreach work for a few months, I met my first dog after Kenneth's Prince. I was walking through Charing Cross Underground when I saw a poor soul sitting in a sleeping bag with a dark brindle Staffie cross. The man looked as if he was in his thirties, and the dog appeared to be quite old, as it had a lovely little grey face and big, wise eyes, which had probably seen a lot over the years.

The man was lost in a different world, clearly an addict in some way, but his arms were clasped around that dog as if she was all he needed, and I could tell by the look in her eyes that she felt exactly the same way. I knew that the man wouldn't engage if I went about it in the wrong way, but I desperately wanted to help him and his fur baby. It was still winter, and he must have been so cold, sitting there in thin clothes, people rushing by never looking at him or his pathetic, worn paper cup which held a few coins.

'Excuse me,' I said, as I got closer, 'could you tell me if this is the right way to get the train to Ealing?' I'd just pulled any place out of my head. I had no idea if it was even the right line, but I needed to find a way to start some kind of conversation with him, as I could sense he might not respond well to someone trying to engage him.

He raised his head ever so slightly and tried to focus, his blue eyes clouded.

'No idea, love,' he muttered, his voice hoarse. 'No idea.'

'Oh, never mind, I'm sure I'll work it out,' I chattered brightly, but he had slumped back into his own little place, not looking at me any longer – but the dog kept her eyes fixed on mine. There was tail-wagging going on too, which was all the encouragement I needed to try again.

'Your dog is gorgeous,' I told him as I squatted down and started an ear scratch on the beautiful creature. 'Is it a boy or a girl?'

The man had a hint of a smile on his face as he looked down at his dog. 'She's a girl,' he said, hugging her even closer as she wagged her tail contentedly. 'She's the best girl in the world – aren't you, Boo?'

'Boo! That's a lovely name,' I replied, but any focus I'd had from him was gone, lost again in his own world, whether because of drink or drugs. Boo was still happily accepting my attention, though, those wise old eyes never leaving mine. 'I'll be back,' I whispered to her. And I was true to my word, returning to Boo and her human every night.

I'd try to engage him, but it was hopeless. It took a week before he even grunted that his name was Callum.

Do you need anything?

No.

Does Boo need anything?

No.

Can I bring you anything tomorrow?

No.

I'm nothing if not determined, though. Callum might be speaking as little as possible, but Boo had been friendly from the first moment I saw her, and she was now beside herself with happiness any time she saw me walking down the Underground tunnel towards them both. I desperately wanted to jump in and help get them both all the things they obviously needed, but I had to wait until Callum had engaged with me and learned that he could trust me. For that, I needed to be patient and consistent, and not put any pressure on him.

Slowly, it began to work. He accepted a scarf, gloves, a flask of tea, soup, things for Boo such as treats and a new collar, a lead, a blanket. As the weeks went by, Callum slowly started to open up to me, little by little, though I never pressed him to tell me anything more than he was comfortable with. He told me of his mental health issues, his drug addiction, the fact that his whole world had collapsed after he had been evicted and that all he had was beautiful Boo. I'd cuddle and kiss her while we talked, and she was very pleased with all of the attention.

Although Callum had finally taken things from me, there was very little I could do for him in terms of the bigger picture. He just wanted a friend to trust and someone he could turn to when needed. It was Callum and Boo who started me on the path of asking around, seeing what there was for pairings like them – owners and dogs who relied on each other and would never be parted. To my shock, the answer seemed to be that there was very little at all. Services just wouldn't accept dogs, and people like Callum wouldn't give up their dogs for love nor money.

There had to be something I could do, and the interaction with Callum and Boo made me think that keeping dogs and owners together was key if these people were ever going to be able to rebuild their lives. I knew how much my own pets meant to me, and I would do anything to keep them by my side, no matter what.

When I wasn't on outreach, or dealing with my own business and family, I was cooking for all the homeless people I came across. I just wanted to be out there supporting them all the time. Dogs were few and far between back then; there were maybe five in the whole area I covered with my street outreach. I'd just help whoever I came across first, taking doggy bits too as I walked Oxford Street, Tottenham Court Road and Leicester Square.

I got to know the dogs much more quickly than some of the people as there was instant trust – and I remembered what they were all called easily too! I got them all leads embroidered with their names – Paddy had a white Staffie called Jazz, and his son Patrick had a brindle Staffie called Gerard, while Damo (who was Paddy's brother and Patrick's uncle) had a tan Staffie called Gypsy. Staffies were certainly the favoured breed of street people. Patrick and Paddy stuck together, and bedded down together, but Damo liked his own company with Gypsy.

There was also Nigel, who had another Staffie, this one called Sketch, and Michael had Lucky. You'll have guessed that Lucky was a Staffie too! I became very close to all of them, getting to know a lot about street dogs and I loved it.

The conversation was more free-flowing with dogs, given that it was only coming from one side, and they just listened to any nonsense that came out of my mouth! I soon discovered that street dogs adore a fuss and they're incredibly sociable. They were icebreakers too. It was easy to ask, 'Do you need anything for the dog? A coat? Food?' and people were much more willing to take something for their dogs than they were for themselves.

At that time, about seven years ago, I was the first one on the streets of Westminster looking after the dogs. My first passion had always been animals and it allowed trust to build up more easily. I'd feel honoured if anyone let me look after their dog if they needed to go somewhere for a moment – I knew how much these dogs meant to their owners, and it was a privilege to be trusted with the responsibility of caring for these beloved creatures, even for a moment, and I was pleased to find that it was becoming more and more common, as people got to know me and I gained their trust.

I never ceased to be amazed at the ways in which homeless people put their animal's needs above their own. They would always choose to feed their dogs before they fed themselves, so I started to educate myself on the nutritional needs of the animals. The problem was, if any homeless person was given food, understandably they wanted to share it with their dog. The result was a lot of the pooches were really fat, being given the completely wrong diets. I tried to gently suggest that they shouldn't just give them pizza or Chinese takeaway leftovers, but soon it became clear that many of the owners couldn't really access proper food.

This became another of my tasks. I'd make up containers of wet food, dry food, nutritious treats, everything that a dog needed to be healthy.

Homeless people have a huge desire for sugar to get that high – it becomes another addiction for them – and they were giving their dogs a lot of the same rubbish. I knew this was something I could address and educate people on, and I made sure that I always had packs of good options and treats wherever I went.

There were very few professional beggars back then, it was mainly only people in genuine need leading raw, rough lives. I started to pick up on the patterns that showed me that someone wasn't faking it, and what I learned then holds good to this day. Genuine rough sleepers are gone by 6 a.m., as lorries come in to deliver stock, the street cleaners also come in at that time and get rid of them, and they leave with their bags of possessions, returning to the same place that night. If someone has nothing with them during the day while they beg, you have to wonder where they have left it – it's more likely that they're faking it.

I became very close to Patrick, Paddy and Damo, as well as their gorgeous dogs, Gerard, Gypsy and Jazz. Paddy's wife – Patrick's mum – had died in Ireland and it all went downhill after she passed, which led to Patrick and Paddy coming to London. Things hadn't worked out for them at all, and they were living a really difficult life with only their dogs to give them the energy to face each day. Damo had always been on the streets, or that was what he told me, and he was a slightly harder character to get to know as he was a bit of a loner.

'If you could have anything, Damo, what would it be?' I asked him one evening.

'A guitar,' he told me in a flash. 'A guitar – and jam sandwiches.'

I had to laugh – I couldn't remember him ever being so quick with an answer before, which had to mean something. 'All right then – I'll be your fairy godmother. A guitar and jam sandwiches will be yours!'

I asked around my friends and acquaintances for a guitar, and was delighted when someone donated an old one their son had long stopped playing. The jam sandwiches were far more straightforward to source! Then I came up with the idea of having a little gathering in Leicester Square where I could give Damo the guitar. I only expected Paddy, Patrick and Damo to come along, with Lucky, Gerard and Gypsy of course, but a few others turned up too. They came into our little group cautiously, as the jam sandwiches were passed round.

When we presented Damo with his guitar, he was utterly lost for words, but from the grin on his face, I could tell he was delighted. He marvelled at it for a while, not saying anything, but then he began strumming, and he was brilliant. It was lovely to watch him play, and everyone stood around, listening and chatting. I felt so content at that moment.

Again, it was proof that the homeless never demand anything. The most important thing to these people is to be acknowledged. That party was a magical moment. The dogs all knew each other anyway, and they just wandered about, wagging their tails, getting far too many treats and a whole lot of attention. I loved that sense of community and it emphasised to me just how much beauty there was in simple things.

I was thrilled one day when Patrick actually did ask for something. It was incredibly unusual, and I couldn't help but feel pleased that it was evidence of a growing bond and the development of some trust between us.

'Michelle . . .' he said quietly, while the others were having some warm soup. 'I've got a huge favour to ask you. I'm so sorry, but I don't know who else to ask. Just say no if it's too much, I'll understand, but I've got nowhere else to turn.' The poor man looked so embarrassed and I geared myself up. I would help if possible, but I knew that what I could do was limited.

'Go on,' I told him. 'Honestly, you can ask me for anything, about anything, and if I can do it, I will.'

He drew breath as if this was something that he needed a lot courage for. 'Do you think that, maybe if there is someone getting rid of a warm coat sometime, you could bear me in mind?'

He looked so ashamed and embarrassed, he could barely meet my eyes, and my heart went out to this young man.

A warm coat. That was what he had been working up towards, the most basic of things. I grabbed my bag and shouted to him, 'I'll be back in fifteen minutes!' and ran to the nearest Primark. I rummaged through the rails until I found the perfect coat. It was waterproof but thick and padded, and would help keep him warm against the elements.

I hurried back to the group and handed Patrick the coat, hoping he would like it. His face lit up at the sight of a brand-new coat, and he hugged me so tightly, it was as if he'd been given the moon. He told me that it was for his dog, Gerard, to cuddle into as well during those cold nights that seemed never-ending, and I couldn't help but think that if he had brought the dog into it from the start, I'd have been even faster off my feet!

Back then, fewer than a quarter of rough sleepers had dogs, so it was still more unusual than not to see them. I used to get very excited if there was a dog around.

I came to be known as the Street Auntie to them all and I could swear that the dogs would smell me from miles away, if their wagging tails were anything to go by. I provided coats, food, collars, leads, all of the essentials, but lots of treats too, and the nutritious food that I knew was so important. On top of that, I had to find money to pay vets' bills, as many of them needed treatments that their owners could never afford. This was a huge outlay, but I also discovered very quickly that street dogs had an incredible survival instinct. We'd panic and get them to the vet as if the world was on fire, while they took it all in their stride, content with a belly rub and a bit of a fuss.

Although I was still working full time alongside my outreach work, and juggling home and family life, I had the amazing feeling that I had woken up to a whole world of new friends. Very quickly I became a safety net for the these people and their dogs, which came in all sizes, shapes, nationalities and breeds. I remember people through their dogs – I might not know who Charles is, but I'll remember Ginger!

There was one pair who really stood out to me in the early days. Ronnie was quite a young man, maybe in his mid-twenties, and he was an avid reader. He was such a lanky lad and it seemed as though he almost had to fold himself up when he was sitting on the streets or cosying up for the night. His dog was some sort of mixed breed called Rover. I used to laugh at that.

'Could you not have thought of something a bit more original, Ronnie?' I joked with him when we first became friends.

'Ah, you're wrong there, Michelle,' he teased. 'Think about it – dogs are all Tallulah this and Lord Fancy Pants that. When did you last hear about a good, solid Rover? It's unusual now, you know – he's a trendsetter, aren't you boy?'

Rover was a massive dog, a bit like his owner, all legs and goofiness. I think there might have been a bit of Lurcher in there, but who knows? A lot of street dogs are Staffies, but many of them are just real Heinz 57 types, and Rover was definitely one of those. He always looked like he had a smile on his face, and was so laid-back, just like his owner. The thing that made Ronnie stand out most though, was that no matter where he was, he'd have a book in his hand and a pile of them in his rucksack. He'd check bins to see if anyone had thrown one away – *how could you do that, how could you throw a book away?* he would wonder – and would regularly scour boxes outside second-hand shops as sometimes they had free titles they would give away if they were damaged. I'm not really one for books, but even I could see that Ronnie was a voracious reader. It was hard to keep him going. He particularly loved thrillers by

Martina Cole and would talk about them for as long as I would listen. He'd tell me every plot, every character, he'd memorise bits of dialogue and tell me what a fantastic writer she was.

'I feel like I've read all of them myself,' I used to say to him.

'I can't do them justice, Michelle – masterpieces they are, masterpieces,' he'd reply and then go off on another lecture about just how brilliant they were. Ronnie didn't have all of her books as he just had to take what he found. I'd pick up any I saw in charity shops, but she's written a lot and he had a fair number of gaps in his portable library.

I had an idea.

When I got home that night – late as always – I switched on my laptop and googled Martina Cole. I found out who her agent was and her publisher, and sent off an email to both just telling them a little bit about Ronnie and how much he loved her, and cheekily asked if there was any chance that they could maybe send him a spare book?

They did more than that! A package arrived about a week later and not only were there all the books he was missing, but Martina Cole had personally signed one for him!

'I've got something for you,' I told him on our next meeting. Rover started jumping up and down – he was about the same height as me when he put his massive paws on my shoulder with excitement – and Ronnie was just as excited. When I gave him the books, I could see the tears well up in his eyes, and the signed one made him feel so important. I'll never forget that gesture – it meant the world to him.

It was these little things that mattered, little things that just said *you're important, you're just as deserving as anyone else*. My time on the streets had only just started, but I was already immersed in the thoughts, lives and feelings of all these wonderful people and their incredible dogs. I knew that there would be much more to learn, however. With the acceptance they had so openly given me, I was up for the challenge.

SIX

All the Fur Babies

I was both mesmerised and shocked by how well these street dogs adapted. The relationship with their owners was amazing. It was like an unbreakable bond. None of them were on leads, they were that obedient – they would never dream of straying away from their owner, no matter what.

Every time I met someone with a dog, I was always told the same thing: 'Michelle, I didn't rescue that dog, the dog rescued me.' I could see that was true, and that the love between them was as pure as anything I had ever come across in my life.

Services for homeless people didn't acknowledge the dogs at all; they were very single-minded in their approach to dealing with individuals. I couldn't help but feel frustrated at the lack of flexibility, but it was nothing compared to the determination of someone on the streets who would fight to stay with their dog at all costs.

As time went by, and as I started to learn more and more about individuals and their lives, I began to see a pattern starting to emerge. The vast majority of homeless men are there because of relationship breakdowns. The dog is theirs already and, when they leave, they take it with them. The dog provides them with a reason to go on, encourages them not to give up. Those without dogs often have a very different outlook, with not as much purpose, I could tell that very easily. If I saw ten homeless people, I'd go to the one with a dog – I could tell that the ones without a dog got more from the services as they moved on quicker. There was no accommodation that took dogs, so if an owner refused to leave their animal, they would be left on the street. I treated everyone I met in the same way, though, and tried to help in whatever way I could. I still had my toy business so they were inundated with dog toys, and I was trying to improve their diets whenever I could as there were too many podgy pups around.

The dogs all seemed so chilled amongst the hustle and bustle, the sirens and noises of life in Central London. A lot of the homeless people I met had ongoing medical conditions, but they couldn't even visit a GP as the dog had nowhere to go, so I'd sit in the car with it. I'd do that if they went to get showers, or had appointments at the hospital. Wherever and whenever they needed me to look after their dog, I'd be there.

This went on for two years. During that time, the council became aware of me. I got the sense that they didn't really want me out there doing my work and pointing out what was wrong with the system, but after a while they realised that they often needed me, as I had a good engagement with with the rough sleepers. I felt like a bit of an outcast at times, if I'm honest; there was a barrier between me and the services, which I guess is how the homeless often felt too.

I wasn't an idiot; I knew there were some scammers out there and I could see the signs. By this point, I reckon one in five were professional beggars. It had taken time to work out what the clues were – I can tell easily now as I know everyone and have the experience, but for a lot of people, the worry of not knowing if someone is being honest or just trying to scam them means that they also don't help those genuinely in need. Let me give you a few pointers.

It's rare for street people to beg as there are many soup kitchens, local food places and humanitarian hand-outs that often look after the rough sleepers. The teams get to know them, and they will give basic help. There are other signs such as the state of their hands and what sort of belongings they have. Someone who is homeless often won't have have clean hands and tidy nails; although there are services through which some people can access showers, this isn't always possible, and that means that the dirt can become ingrained. Similarly, if they're sitting begging, they will have all their worldly goods with them if their need is real. Genuine homeless people don't just sit at cash machines, waiting and begging; they actually prefer to stay hidden, to remain invisible to avoid all the judgement they get.

People don't understand that there is a parallel world out there. It's happening right under our noses, but if you don't look, it is easy to have no idea at all. Tragically, there are many, many homeless people who die on the streets or in hostel accommodation every day, every week and every month, and there is an annual commemoration service to remember them held at an event in November at St Martin's-in-the-Fields Church at Trafalgar Square.

The memorial service is an opportunity to acknowledge the passing of these poor souls, many of whom won't have had a proper funeral service, and some who don't even have any family or friends to know that they have passed. It breaks my heart that someone could die without a single person in the world to care.

I first heard about this memorial service through the grapevine, and it was in 2014 that I went to my first one. It was a beautifully crisp but bitterly cold day, with sunlight streaming through the stained-glass windows. There was an incredible juxtaposition between the beauty and wealth of such a place and the type of congregation they had that day. Although there were social workers and people who worked with homeless charities, in each pew sat row after row of rough sleepers – and their dogs.

When I walked in, the coldness of the air hit me and I was glad that I had worn my warmest quilted coat; so many of those around me were denied that luxury. They were in their street clothes, of course, no full wardrobe for them to choose from depending on the weather, and there was a stark brutality in how exposed they were. The only people I could see wearing scarves and hats were those I knew – and I had given them those things at the start of winter. For me, there was a treat afterwards – I'd promised myself a hot drink and some cake in a toasty café – whereas the homeless people here would only get that if I took it to them. Which, of course, I would.

The minister gave a lovely reading and spoke of those who had passed that year. The list was far too long. If it had only comprised of one name, it would have been too long. To hear those words, to hear of those lives unnecessarily lost, chilled me to the bone even more than the winter temperature in the church that day. It was a very subdued atmosphere and I'm sure that a great number of those attending were heartbroken as they reflected on those they had lost. It wouldn't be a huge stretch of the imagination to guess that they were also thinking of their own fates as they sat there with their dogs, listening to another year's list of names being read out. A lot of rough sleepers go to the service every year, perhaps to mark that they're still surviving. It is a social thing to some extent, a reason to connect for a little while.

When it ended, so many people came up to me and asked, 'Are you Michelle? Are you the lady who helps the dogs?' It was lovely to know that word was spreading, and that people must have been speaking to each other about the help I was providing.

They certainly shouldn't have had any concerns about whether I respected and cared for the homeless and their dogs. After so long not quite knowing what I was doing, or what my purpose was, I truly felt that this was my calling. Homeless people are beautiful souls. What I find so wonderful about them is that they are very straightforward. They have nothing to prove, and they feel like they have nothing to lose.

I'm like that too. What you see is what you get. If you like it, great; if you don't, fine. I can be myself around the homeless. I don't need a rulebook or tick boxes, or terms and conditions, and that gets me a connection with them much more quickly. I don't let them down and that consistency means the world to them. They need to have control and not be dictated to. If they think they've failed, that's a disaster. I deal with a multitude of complex issues out there and everyone has a story to tell, but it has to be in their own time and on their own terms.

The dogs have their own ways too. Street dogs suffer greater anxiety than dogs who live inside. They need to protect both their owner and themselves, and monitor the whole environment around them constantly. When they first live on the street, it is startling to them, but they do adapt if they're with someone who loves them. And there is a lot of love out there. For a rough sleeper, their dog is their everything. The dog often stops them ending their lives because they feel they have a huge responsibility to the dog and it can save them, but they feel guilty too for giving them that sort of life. None of those dogs should be on the streets, but neither should the people. I often see old dogs sleeping rough, and it does make me sad to think of them ending their years without a soft bed in a warm house, but I also know that they would have more trauma if they were parted, so great is the attachment to their owner. Each pair is deeply tuned into each other's feelings and needs, and the bond is extremely powerful, often in a way that doesn't exist with indoors dogs, where some owners see their pets as nothing more than fashion accessories, or get walkers in to look after them most of the time and never really engage with the dogs.

In some ways, there is no typical day in the life of a street dog because of the strange mix of the mundane and unpredictable, which their owners experience too. Some days are the same as the hundred before, with only the weather changing, but others can be dramatic or terrifying. In a usual day, however, there are things which never change, no matter the dog. There is a lot of walking about for them all. It's exercise, but not in the way our dogs would have. There's a freedom to our dogs' lives that street dogs just don't have. They're always by their owner's side and their day revolves around them.

For dogs who have loving homes with us, there will be a routine: morning walk, evening walk, that last toilet of the evening. They will have their two meals a day, they'll have their cosy bed, their favourite spot by the fire or on the sofa, they'll have treats they go nuts for, and a toy that sends them wild with happiness. A street dog has no such routine because their owner has no routine – the dog is very much on the timetable of the person, but that notion of a 'timetable' is pretty loose every day anyway; sometimes it can be nothing more than daytime and night-time.

The lack of routine affects the behaviour of these dogs. When our dogs run off, we chase after them screaming blue murder, terrified they'll belt over a road or disappear with no sense to somewhere they've never been to before. Not street dogs. They always, *always* have the owner in sight. They're the most obedient, well-trained dogs you could ever meet. Sometimes, they're not so sociable with other dogs, but they are fantastic with people. They do have some anxiety, that's true, but this is because they need to protect themselves and their owners above all else, and, because of that, they lead quite self-isolating lives.

They are special dogs – they sit there or walk without leads quite often – while the bustle of the city never stops. Fire engines, police cars, all the sirens and wailing just goes over their heads and they focus, focus, focus on their owner. That is all they care about, all that matters. Sometimes, though, there is a dog who goes beyond even those amazing things, a dog who saves the life of their owner.

One such dog was Doris. I adored that name, and I adored Doris from the moment we met. Her owner, Billy, had recognised me from the remembrance service where we'd met briefly, and cheerily shouted, 'Hello there!' next time I was out on the street walking around, looking to see if everyone was OK or if there was anyone new who I hadn't come across before.

'Hi!' I grinned at him, 'How are you?'

'Oh fine, fine, you know how it is, can't complain,' he replied.

He had plenty to complain about from what I could see, but he clearly had a positive attitude. Billy was a very thin man, middle-aged, with a strong Scottish accent. But Doris – oh Doris! She was a fluffy little black terrier, who dashed about from him to me and back again as if she had all the energy in the world and couldn't wait to run some of it off!

Her dad was full of energy too, and very chatty. 'I saw you at that service,' he told me, 'and people were saying how much you help dogs.' I nodded. 'That's how you tell whether someone is a good person. If you like dogs, I like you.'

'Can't argue with that!' I laughed.

'Funny place this, though,' he went on, waving his arm

around. 'I was at that service to try and make a few pals as it's been a bit lonely since I arrived here with Doris. You ever been to Scotland?'

'No, no I haven't – I'd love to though. It's meant to be very beautiful.'

'Oh aye – all castles and lochs, and tartan and haggis, and Glasgow, where I'm from, well, it's the best place in the world,' he winked. 'Not for me though. It's not for me now.' There was such sadness in his eyes then, and Doris had calmed now, sensing his mood and just sitting quietly by his side.

'I'm from Glasgow, did I mention that?' I nodded. 'God, I miss it,' he continued. 'I was brought up in the East End district, maybe not the most glamorous place in the world, but the friendliest, definitely the friendliest.' He grinned cheekily. 'And there are plenty who would fight you if you said otherwise! Maybe I'll get back there though, maybe one day.'

'I'm sure you will,' I said, comfortingly, 'it's not that far on the train, is it?'

'No, no, not at all. That's how we got here actually. Me and my little stowaway here. I hid her in my bag and she pretty much slept the whole way.'

I wondered how someone who had afforded the train ticket from Glasgow to London had ended up on the streets. I should have known even from our short time together that Billy wasn't one for holding back on his story.

'I bet you've heard every tale under the sun, haven't you, Michelle?'

'I've heard a few.'

'Mine was army, ex-army now, I guess. Got back from service and life just seemed a bit tricky really. Going to the supermarket, cutting the grass, playing with the kids, all the normal stuff, then the flashbacks, the stuff you don't really want. Bit hard to combine it all,' he said, which was an understatement to say the least. 'You see things when you are in that job and nothing can prepare you for it. There are men who seem like the strongest in the world at the start, who end up crumbling. There are others who find it the making of them. I think I was a wee bit in both camps. My dad and my brothers were all military – it runs through our blood for generations. Plenty of Scots like that though, there's not much of an option in some places. I always assumed I'd join up – but I guess I always thought it would be plain sailing. My dad never mentioned what he had been through, but I wonder now – I wonder what he saw over all those years. It felt like where I was meant to be an awful lot of the time, Michelle. You make pals there who understand it all, you see, and you bond like nothing else on earth.

'Then, you come back. Just for a wee while to start with, and you're that pleased. Fair away with yourself, as us Scots would say. Then one day, the telly seems too loud, the bairns a bit annoying even though they're only playing, the wife going on about something that – excuse my French – you couldn't give a shit about, and you realise you're missing it. You want to go back.'

'It must be so hard,' I sympathised. 'Always going from one place to the next, on tour then back home.'

'Aye, it is. And then, once I'd left, once I was told I had no choice but to leave, I was lost. My family couldn't really understand, though. They just wanted the old Billy back. And the more I felt on my own with it all, the more I felt I *should* be on my own with it all. I got this little one to try and make me feel a bit more like myself. Thought that the walking would help, thought that she would do the trick.'

'And has she?' I asked, deliberately not prying into why Billy had been asked to leave the army.

'Aye, for a wee bit. But then it was as if it was just me and her against the world. She was with me all the time. I wasn't working, I'd left the army on medical grounds, and we had all the time in the world together, didn't we, Doris?'

That little terrier adored Billy, it was plain to see. She stared at him all through his story and he never took his hand off her, scratching and tickling her behind the ears.

'Anyway, I've taken up enough of your time, droning on – I'm sure you've got better things to do.'

I hadn't really. It was getting dark, but being here with them was what I wanted. However, I could tell Billy had said all he wanted, so I took his cue and stood up.

'Is there anything I can get for you or Doris?' I asked.

'I suppose a wee dram's out of the question?' he laughed.

'I'm afraid so – strict no "'wee dram" policy here! Do you need something to eat, does Doris need anything?'

'No, nothing for me, I'm fine, not hungry at all – but maybe a treat for Doris would be nice.'

I was back with Billy and Doris the next night, and the next, and the next. More of his story came out. He spun a good tale and I loved his accent, which made it a pleasure to sit there, cuddling Doris and listening. Billy had received a decent payout from the army when he left. He never told me what his medical condition was, which made me wonder whether that hadn't been the real reason and he was just hiding that part of his history, which was entirely his prerogative. Once he'd left the army, he moved back home permanently to Glasgow with his wife and kids, as he'd said, but things just didn't fall into place. Life on Civvy Street was harder than on military tour. Constant arguing with his wife had led to things being said that could never be unsaid, and the lack of any sort of mental health support made him feel that there was no option but to leave. Starting a new life in London was going to be his saving grace. He'd do well, sort himself out, then go back to his wife Louise to fix their marriage.

Billy had enough money to stay somewhere for a couple of weeks while he got on his feet, but he couldn't find anywhere centrally that was affordable and that would take dogs.

'It's funny,' he said, 'I see all these posh women coming out of fancy hotels with wee dogs in their handbags just like Doris, and that's fine, they get to do that – but us? No, we're not wanted even in the cheap places, are we, Doris?'

I could have spent all my spare time with those two. I loved his stories and he was so open about everything, which was quite unusual, and it made me really appreciate his trust in me. He never wanted anything substantial, always said he wasn't hungry, and would only take water or his favourite diet drinks. I didn't know why – he could have had sugary ones all day as he was so skinny. In fact, he looked as if he was losing weight from one day to the next.

Doris loved all of her treats though, and I'd given her a little rubber ball to play with. She'd push it away from her with her tiny black nose then race after it on her ridiculously short legs before bringing it back to us and doing it all over again. Billy worshipped her and didn't really seem to have made any friends amongst the other rough sleepers, although they always said 'hello' to each other.

I'd been spending a lot of time with Billy and Doris, and so, one day, a few weeks after we'd met, I went to the bench where he often sat. It was earlier than we usually met, but even though it was daytime, I was surprised to find that Billy was fast asleep, Doris curled up at his feet. He was completely conked out, and for a horrible moment, I wasn't certain that he was breathing. I gave him a little nudge just to check he was OK, and to my relief, he let out a small groan, though he didn't wake up.

I had never smelled alcohol off Billy, and he'd only asked for that 'wee dram' the once (and even that was through mischief, I thought), but when I finally roused him, his voice was slurred and he couldn't manage to sit up.

'Billy, are you sure you're OK?' I asked, feeling worried.

'Aye, aye, I'm fine,' he said weakly, his thinning red hair plastered to his skull.

'What can I get you? A sandwich? Burger?'

'No, no – maybe just a bottle of water, or two if that's OK. I'm just a bit warm, that's all.'

When I got back with his water a few minutes later, Billy had fallen asleep again. There were two other rough sleepers I knew nearby.

'Michelle!' one of them shouted over, waving a greeting. 'That bloke doing all right?'

'I think so – maybe. I'm not sure. He seems really tired. Have you been speaking to him today?'

'Not really,' said the older of the two. 'He was here when we arrived and he's been flat out since then. The dog's watching him, but I think he must have taken something as he's been dead to the world this whole time.'

I nodded. Something wasn't right.

'Keep an eye on him when you can, will you boys?'

'Sure, sure we will,' they promised, and I reluctantly headed off. Before I went, I gently bent down to ensure

Billy was still breathing. He was, but there was a terrible smell coming off his breath that made me question all that I'd ever thought of him. My heart sank at the realisation that Billy had succumbed to one of the addictions of the street. He'd definitely been drinking – a large amount, judging by the state of him – and I wondered just how fast he would go down this terrible path, and what it would mean for him and Doris.

SEVEN

Doris Saves the Day

In the short time I'd known Billy, I'd grown to really like him. He was gentle and funny, he had opened up to me quickly, and his dog was adorable. However, the streets were cruel. Who knows how horrible his demons were or what he had been battling? Perhaps he had addictions before he ever got to London, perhaps he'd been here for much longer than he'd said. I could only take the stories as they were given to me, and I could only do what was within my power.

I thought about Billy and Doris all day and all night. I barely slept that night, and woke up at the crack of dawn the next morning. I decided to go back to the part of the city where I always saw them and try to get to Billy before he had his next drink or fix. The sun was rising by the time I parked, and I half walked, half ran to where I knew, or at least hoped, Billy would be.

I could hear the whimpering before I even got there.

Doris!

My stomach lurched as I dreaded to think what I might find.

It was just as bad as I'd anticipated. Billy was lying there on the ground, completely comatose, with Doris squealing at his feet. The poor little dog was clearly terrified, repeatedly pawing at him with no effect.

'Billy! Billy!' I shouted, but there was no point. He was out of it, and the smell that was coming from him was horrendous, I wondered if it might even be turps. I quickly pulled my phone out of my pocket and dialled 999, giving them exact details of where we were and Billy's state. I also told them that I was an outreach worker in the hope that wouldn't simply dismiss this as 'just' a homeless person. To their credit, they were there within minutes. Doris was distraught, and I tried to soothe her but she was shaking and whining as she tried desperately to try to get back to her beloved owner.

The paramedics were loading Billy into the ambulance when I got to it.

'Can I come with him?' I asked.

'Not unless you're family,' I was told.

'It was me who found him, and I really need to know that he'll be OK.'

'Sorry love, we can't just let anyone come.'

'I found him! I'm an outreach worker and I've been talking to him every day for over a week. I know lots about him,' I said, hoping I could hook them in with the promise of being able to fill out some forms, which wasn't strictly true.

The two paramedics looked at each other before one said, 'Well, we can't stop you following us, can we?'

That was all I needed. The car was parked nearby so I scooped Doris up into my arms and ran to get it. Just as I was leaving, I spoke to the paramedic who was hooking Billy up to a drip after she'd taken a blood finger prick. 'It looks bad, doesn't it? Drugs or alcohol, do you think?'

She looked at me as if I was daft.

'It's not drugs or alcohol, it's ketones,' she said. 'You can smell the ketones off him a mile away. He's in a diabetic coma and we just need to get him stabilised on some insulin as his blood sugar is through the roof.'

Diabetic! I'd had no idea Billy was diabetic. I felt terrible for thinking that he was drunk, or using, when in fact he urgently needed medical treatment for his illness. I just prayed that the paramedics would get him to hospital in time.

I sped through the streets, following the ambulance as closely as I could, and hurried to find a parking space, desperately hoping that Billy would be OK. As I hurried into the A&E department, I pleaded with the receptionist on the front desk to give me some information about Billy, or the state he was in, but as I wasn't a family member, she refused to give me any more information.

She could obviously tell I was distraught, so she told me to come back during visiting hours the next day. Reluctantly I left, unable to bear the thought of having to wait to get the rest of Billy's story.

I went home feeling exhausted and incredibly shaken, but desperate to know more. To my relief, Doris had calmed down a little by now, and settled down at my feet. I had no idea what had really happened to Billy. I googled 'diabetes' and 'ketones' and the more I read about the illness, the more I found so many things that made sense when I thought of how Billy had been acting. There are two kinds of diabetes, with the first, Type 1, needing insulin. Type 2 can be controlled by diet and/or tablets, but it seemed to me that Billy must have Type 1. If diabetics don't keep their blood sugars at a stable level, then they spiral out of control and they get ketones in their blood. If this goes on too long, it's life-threatening. Like Billy, they can fall into a diabetic coma, and even die if there is no treatment forthcoming. To do everything necessary in order to stay healthy with diabetes whilst living on the streets would be almost impossible.

The next day, I left Doris with a close friend and I raced to the hospital to be there as soon as visiting hours began. Billy was still on a drip, but sitting up, looking clean and far healthier than the last time I'd seen him, though he still looked exhausted, and far too thin.

'Well, you gave me a bit of a fright, didn't you?' I joked, as if telling him off, but he only had one thing on his mind.

'Doris. Where is she? Is she OK? Do you know who has her? Please tell me she's safe.'

'It's fine, it's fine – please don't worry, Billy. She was the one who let me know there was something wrong with you in the first place. She came home with me last night and she's in safe hands, don't you worry. I'll look after her until you're better and make sure she gets plenty of treats and food. Honestly, she'll be fine until you get back on your feet. You need to focus on getting yourself better, for your sake as well as Doris's. You really did worry me, Billy.'

We spent the rest of the visiting hours talking about what had happened to him – it wasn't as if anyone else was going to turn up for a chat with Billy.

'I guess you know the whole story now?' Billy asked, looking at me sadly.

I would never presume to know someone's story in its entirety, so I merely said, 'I'm a good listener.'

'Aye – I bet you are, I bet you hear some things! The thing is, Michelle, I'd been feeling a bit rough for a while. Thirsty all the time, losing weight, absolutely knackered, so when I went for one of the routine checks we get, I mentioned this. One wee prick of the finger later and they said I had diabetes. My blood sugar was through the roof and they didn't know how I was even still standing. The only thing that was maybe helping to keep the blood sugar down a bit was all the exercise I did as that affects it.

'They told me I was Type 1 – it's usually Type 2 at my age, and often folk who are a bit on the, shall we say, tubby side, but not me. I was in the group where I couldn't stay in the army any longer. It would be a daily routine of blood tests and insulin injections for the rest of my life, so I left. When I got home, it wasn't just the change from the army that I had to deal with – I now had a life-changing condition that needed constant monitoring. It's possible to live a normal life with diabetes, but it takes a lot of hard work and commitment, which could never be done when I worked in something which had no predictability at all. Maybe I could have gone into office work in the army but that would never have worked. Not for me.

'I felt that I was a burden on everyone. There had been too much change all at once, and I just wanted to get away from it all.'

He did have money; he'd been telling the truth about the payout he'd got from leaving the army, but he only took a small portion of it to get him and Doris to London, with a little extra for the short time he thought it would take him to make a new life. He left the rest for his wife and kids. He hadn't planned for it to be forever, he just needed to find his feet.

'I had no idea how hard it would be,' he told me. 'You get this little meter to test your blood sugars every day – but it isn't once, it isn't even twice, it's before every meal and at other times if you feel your blood is too high or too low. You have to inject insulin into your legs or your arms or your tummy or your bum before every meal, and you have to constantly be aware of your food, your exercise, so many things.'

'How could you be expected to manage all that on the streets though, Billy?' I asked. 'No wonder it all got too much, especially when it was new to you.'

'I had this idea,' he said. 'You take insulin to balance out the amount of food you eat, but if you don't have enough food, or too much insulin, or too much exercise, you go hypo. When you're hypo, you can collapse as your blood sugar drops too low. I couldn't risk that. I never knew when I would get food, and I was walking around all day, so I thought I would try the other option. If I didn't have insulin, and I didn't eat, then I thought my blood would stay stable. That's why I never took food from you.'

'And that's why you always wanted diet coke or water?' I asked.

'Aye – but also, when your blood sugar is too high, you get a raging thirst on you because you have these ketones. You're completely dehydrated because of the acid in your body and you just can't get enough water to stop it.'

'And they smell? These ketones smell?'

'Oh aye, they stink!'

'I thought it was booze or turps,' I told him.

'Some folk say it's like peardrop sweeties, but it's definitely a smell you notice,' he agreed. 'I'd been warned, when the doctor was telling me how to manage my diabetes, that a lot of folk just think you're drunk, whether your blood is too high or too low, as you stumble about and don't really make sense.'

It was all an education to me, and something that has stood me in good stead over the years. After leaving Billy, I checked up on Doris, giving her lots of cuddles and telling her what a good girl she was, and went off on my rounds for the rest of the day and night.

Billy had mentioned to me that as soon as his insulin regime was sorted out in hospital, things would be fine very quickly and he'd be discharged, but I was completely unprepared for what was waiting for me the next day when I went in.

'Michelle!' shouted Billy, who was sitting in a chair, clean as a whistle, and freshly shaven. 'Meet Louise!'

A tiny little, very pretty, dark-haired woman was sitting next to Billy, holding his hand.

'You're Billy's wife!' I declared, my eyes wide with surprise. I remembered Billy telling me her name way back when we first met, but I couldn't imagine how she was there now.

'I certainly am,' she said, smiling up at me, 'and I believe I have a *lot* to thank you for, Michelle.'

'Oh, you're very welcome for all of it – it's been my pleasure. I do have one question though: how did you know he was here?'

'I'm still next of kin on his medical records. I got a phone call when they admitted him to hospital. I was terrified, but it was such a relief to know where he was at long last. I've been worried sick all these months, trying desperately to track him down – I had no idea where he was. I left the kids with my folks and got the first flight I could down from Glasgow. I just can't believe what's he's been through.' She squeezed his hand, her eyes filling with tears.

'Not just ending up in here, but living on the streets, all of that. It stops now, you hear me? It stops now, Billy. We're a family and we'll get through anything and everything together.'

Tears spilled down Billy's cheeks, and I had a lump in my throat as I watched them both together. Billy seemed like such a kind man, and in the short time I'd been working with homeless people, I knew that happy endings like this were all too rare.

As Billy sat there with adoring eyes, nodding along to everything Louise said, it struck me that there wasn't much difference between her and Doris! Both of them tiny and determined, both of them willing to fight and protect Billy, save him from his own self-destruction.

'I suppose I'd better go and collect that silly wee dog of yours before we go, hadn't I?'

'When are you being discharged?' I asked.

'Tomorrow – everything's going really well, and we're getting the train back up tomorrow afternoon so that Doris can come with us.'

'Not hidden in your bag this time, I hope!' I joked with him, as Louise rolled her eyes.

'Really, Billy? You hid that wee dog in a bag?' chastised Louise. 'You do have a lot to tell me, don't you?'

Before I left, I gave Louise my number, telling her to let me know what time they'd be ready to leave the next day. I told them I'd bring Doris with me and then meet them outside the hospital before dropping them all at King's Cross.

I arrived there at 10 a.m., just as planned, and it was like picking up two lovebirds. I'd chatted to Doris the whole way, telling her she would see her daddy soon, but when Billy and Doris were reunited, it was like something out of a love story! The little terrier was beside herself with happiness and I swear a few tears fell from Billy's eyes. He was a changed man – clean, on his way to good health, reunited with his wife, soon to see his family, and, most importantly, back with Doris!

When they got out of my car, Billy leaned back in through my window.

'You have no idea what you've done for me, Michelle,' he said. 'Honestly, you've given me everything back again. But I know that even if I had stayed on the streets, having someone like you there would have made a world of difference. You just keep doing what you're doing – and when you see Harry . . . well, there's no words to thank him for looking after this wee girl really, but I'm sure you'll do it better than I ever could.'

With that, they all walked off, quickly consumed by the crowds of people in the station and, hopefully, to a much better life. I hoped with all my heart that Billy and Doris would have the happiest of lives. They both deserved it so very much. It would have been nice to just sit there and reflect for a while, but a combination of traffic wardens, horn-tooting drivers, and a need to go check on dozens of other rough sleepers brought me back to reality!

Doris had been a brilliant street dog. She may have been small, but she was fiercely protective of Billy and they'd been a good team. She'd learned the ways of the street just as so many had before her, but I was so thankful that she and Billy had been able to leave that life behind them. I knew how rare that was.

I got to know more and more about street people every day. I found out about the services; the whole community. I faced a lot of closed doors, as if I was stepping on their territory. It was intense at times and more dogs were slowly appearing. I started a soup kitchen because rough sleepers didn't always have easy access to good food. When passers-by did give them something, it was usually from a fast-food chain as that was what could be accessed quickly. Things were either pretty unhealthy or processed. What they really needed was nutritious, healthy food that was solid and left them full up for more than five minutes. It was the same problem I had with their dogs actually!

I was buying fresh fruit and veg at supermarkets for them, cooking meals at my own house constantly, and I needed to find a more efficient way of doing it. I set the soup kitchen up in Shoreditch and it was instantly popular, providing yet another option for those who needed things most. I was also going further afield and finding people with such complex needs. Billy had taught me about diabetes but there was one client who had cerebral palsy, another had no legs.

Christmas was always a poignant time for me as it was when I'd first had my eyes opened by Kenneth and Prince outside Waitrose. For those on the street, it was poignant for different reasons – the festive period inevitably brought back memories of the lives left behind, or for others in a position where living on the street was better than what they'd faced at home, it was a reminder of the horrors they had left behind.

For all those living on the streets in the winter, there was no escape from the cold and the rain, the days that seemed to be dark all the time, and the obvious signs of Christmas preparation from other people living ordinary lives, laden down with shopping bags.

I decided that the homeless would have their own Christmas to celebrate this time; to bring some joy to the streets. I'd been doing present boxes for the dogs from the first year, but I now moved on to a party. There were mince pies, panettone, crackers, all the traditional things (apart from alcohol) in a very non-traditional setting. I loved doing it and I felt honoured to gather together with these inspiring people.

Through my work, I was definitely starting to get a name out there. It was becoming clear to everyone, both in my life on the street and my old life, that this wasn't just a hobby or something that I would drop. Rain, snow . . . if they were out in it, I wanted to be beside them. However, it was emotionally draining work and I felt as though I was needed everywhere, at all times. There weren't enough hours in the day, and I couldn't help but sometimes become down at the limitations of what I could do. Anyone I came across, I'd stop the car, but I was frustrated because I couldn't get them off the street. They called me their angel but I just wished I had magic powers to sort it all, make everything perfect, especially for those dogs.

The extent of mental health problems suffered by those living on the streets is awful. Whatever you can think of – bipolar, depression, schizophrenia, eating disorders – it's there. How can people be expected to deal with that, find food, find shelter, look after their dog, as well as formulate a plan to get their lives back on track? They just can't. And there was the perennial problem of accommodation – if you have a dog, you can't come in, and if you have to leave your dog, you lose a part of yourself. It was an impossible position for these people to be in, and I could never get their words out of my mind – *I didn't save my dog, my dog saved me.* Those fur babies carried so much, and they did it with such grace.

Heat and cold are both equally bad for people and animals. There is so much sunstroke amongst those sleeping rough, with people having heat-induced fits.

Water is such a basic human need, but for rough sleepers and their dogs, having regular access to it can be impossible at times. I was horrified to learn that passers-by often assumed that homeless people were sleeping or drunk when in fact they had collapsed as a result of dehydration, which can be deadly.

Dogs can't walk on hot pavements for long – the little pads on their paws blister easily, so I would emphasise that their owners needed to go to shaded areas with them. I'd give them cooling blankets, and sun cream, especially for their noses. Dogs can't sweat so they need to be watched constantly for signs of dehydration. The more time I spent on the streets, the more I learned – even little things proved useful, such as the fact that dogs with white noses burn more easily.

No matter if it was winter or summer, there was always something to do. I'm not suggesting that other people should deny themselves things because of those who have less, but think of how it must feel to someone with nothing as you walk by, enjoying a summer's day without a worry in the world, eating an ice cream that cost you a fiver, shopping for summer clothes, planning a holiday, all without a care in the world.

At Christmas, many people spend hundreds, sometimes thousands, of pounds on gifts that may well be ignored come Boxing Day. There is so much waste out there. I try not to judge, and I would never judge the street sleepers, but I do wish I could just say to some people, *maybe you could spend just a little money on other things, donate to a dog rescue, give someone a blanket or a pair of thick socks.* It isn't my place to say those things, though. I may think it, but I would never say it.

During that period, my days and nights were just a whirlwind of checking up on everyone, making sure the dogs were all right, trying to plan some nice activities to give the dogs and owners something to look forward to. I thought I was at peak capacity at that stage, but, looking back, those were the days when I actually had room to breathe!

EIGHT

Meeting Tom

There are lots of little squares dotted around London, green spaces with trees and grass, corners where someone could sit quietly and be almost hidden, benches where they could rest and perhaps chat – although they can no longer sleep on benches as most of them have had anti-homeless barriers put on them by councils, as if sleep is something else they don't deserve. There are benches that commemorate famous writers or artists, that say who has lived or died nearby, what inventions and books were created in the tall buildings around them, but no attention is paid to the type of life that is now going on inside these squares.

I was walking through one of them, just off a main street, wondering if there was anyone I'd missed. I knew a lot of street sleepers and their dogs by now, but there would always be new people, or some who didn't want to make contact yet. I suddenly thought to myself, *take a couple of minutes to yourself, Michelle; have a sit down and just enjoy the sun for a moment.*

I must have unwittingly closed my eyes for a moment because I was suddenly aware of someone approaching me and I opened my eyes to see a huge bloke standing in front of me. He must have been about six foot four, maybe more, but he was slouched over as if trying to make himself smaller.

'Hello,' I said. 'How are you doing?'

He just nodded back at me, not saying anything, so I held out my hand. 'Nice to meet you,' I smiled. I indicated to the space next to me on the bench and asked him if he wanted to take a load off. He did hesitate, but that isn't unusual. To me, I'd think I was pretty unthreatening, just a middle-aged woman with a lot of bags, probably looking as if I'd been shopping. This fella would have no idea that my bags were full of socks and dog treats, leads and collars. Street people know that attacks, verbal or physical, can come from anyone, anywhere, and someone who may look innocuous can turn quickly to the type who spouts venom at them.

He definitely looked like he was sleeping rough: he was dishevelled, unshaven, carrying even more plastic bags than me, and he had that air of not feeling that he had a right to talk. That was something I noticed so often – the sense among so many of the homeless that they were undeserving, that they needed to be 'allowed' to speak or come closer, or even just be there.

He didn't shake my hand, but he did sit down beside me. I chatted about things that didn't matter – the weather, tourists, stuff like that, when out of nowhere he spoke.

'I saw you last night. With a man. And a dog. You were giving them things.'

'That's what I do,' I laughed. 'I give things to dogs!'

'I want you to help me find someone,' he said, very quietly. He had a strong Irish accent, and the softness of its tone matched the softness of his words. 'I'm looking for another woman. She's called Michelle, and she helps dogs too. Do you know her? Maybe you're friends. I don't know – maybe one woman who helps dogs knows another woman who helps dogs. That could be the way of it.'

I leaned over to him. 'Maybe I'm Michelle,' I said.

The man laughed, a gorgeous, rich belly laugh, and shook his head, 'Well, wouldn't that be grand?'

'It would – and it is.' I reached out my hand again. 'Let's go back to the start. Hello, I'm Michelle.'

He looked at me as if he was dreaming, actually rubbing his eyes before he responded. 'For sure? You're the Michelle I'm looking for?'

'I'm definitely Michelle – whether you're going to be happy with that, I don't know. Is there something I can do to help?'

To my shock, at my words, his whole body started to shudder with sobbing, deep gulps that came from his very soul. He was such a big man and it was heartbreaking to see. Totally broken, there was a weight on his shoulders that I desperately wanted to help him carry, but I knew not to press him for his story, as was my rule – if he wanted to tell me, he would. All I could do was to gently stroke his arm and hand him tissues until he'd got it all out. After a while, the shaking and the sobbing eased a bit.

'Are you really Michelle?' he asked again.

I nodded.

'Can you help me find her? Can you help find my Poppy?'

And there it was. In a flash, although I didn't know it and he didn't know it, Tom had come into my life with the dog who would change my world. Well, the dog I had to find *before* she could change my world.

'I'll do what I can, I promise you that – she *is* a dog isn't she?' I checked, wondering for just a second if maybe I was committing to tracking down a wayward wife or girlfriend! I wouldn't be surprised, given that I never knew what I was going to face.

He laughed for the first time. 'Yeah, yeah! She's a dog – she's the best dog in the world. I'm Tom,' he told me and shook my hand properly for the first time, really pumping it up and down, holding on with the other hand as if his life depended on it. 'I can't believe it's you – I can't believe I've found you when I least expected it.'

'Hold on Tom, you sit there, and I'll go get us a coffee. I've got a feeling we've got a lot of chatting to do. What would you like?'

He looked at me as if I'd offered him the moon.

'Just . . . anything. You don't have to,' he said.

This was common. Being given a choice, being given that little bit of humanity could seem so alien to a person living on the streets that they had to almost be persuaded to take up any offer.

'Coffee? Tea? Sugar? Milk? Cake? Crisps? Water? Orange juice? Sandwich?' I rattled them all off as Tom threw his hands up.

'Whatever! Whatever!' he smiled. 'Honestly, you choose.'

I walked off to the nearest coffee shop, which was no more than a couple of hundred yards away from the little grassy square and I'd only been gone a few steps when Tom called.

'Michelle,' he called. 'To be honest – I do like a cup of milky tea with four sugars and a nice bit of cake. If you're offering, that is,' he winked.

By the time I got back, he was more composed. I took a moment to look at Tom more closely as I walked back to the bench. He was as tall as I had first sensed, slim, and without a single hair on his head. There wasn't even any stubble on it, and it was hard for homeless men to be able to shave regularly, so I guessed it must be alopecia, possibly from the stress of living on the streets.

'You looking at my lovely shiny head there, Michelle?' he smiled. 'I keep it that way so that pretty girls like you can see themselves in it,' he winked. 'Or maybe the fairies took it away when I went into one of their homes without an invitation. Or maybe it's so I can rub it for good luck. Who knows, Michelle? It's certainly not brought me any of that good luck as I've lost my girl, I've lost my Poppy.'

He was going to tip right over into melancholy if I didn't get him back on track. 'Well, why don't you tell me about Poppy?' I said.

'From the beginning?' he asked.

'From wherever you like.'

'Well, she's gone. I've lost her,' Tom said, shaking his head. 'I need you to find her.'

'Where did you lose her?' I knew it was very rare for a street dog to leave its owner's side, and my mind was racing to all the places a dog might be if it had run off; could she be injured, where would she be if that was the case? I definitely needed to know more of this story.

'We've been together so long,' Tom started to open up. 'Before this . . .' he waved his arms around, 'before we ended up with nothing . . . well, I never had "nothing" because I always had her, you know?' I nodded. I did know, and his words reminded me of my own past, and the solace animals had given me. 'It's a long story, but life happens and my life mainly revolved around alcohol for a while.' At this point, nothing shocked me anymore, and I didn't bat an eyelid as he glanced up at me nervously, as though trying to gauge my reaction. People have their histories and it isn't for me to judge. Although it sounded as though alcohol was in his past, I could smell alcohol from his breath and knew that it was likely something that he still struggled with. That said, it was none of my business.

'I got in with some bad people, and I moved away,' he went on. 'Then, I thought I'd hit the jackpot when I fell in love but she had her demons too. Christ, her demons made mine seem like a walk in the park. I had to get out – it was the only way I'd survive. I never lifted a finger to her in all the time we were together – that's not something she could say about what she did to me, though.'

Tom wasn't making eye contact with me as he told me his story. I've no doubt that he was painting himself in a good light; however, letting him talk was what mattered.

'So, I left,' he stated. 'I left. Not alone though – I took Poppy. I would never have gone without her, I love the bones of that dog and whatever life I was heading towards, I wanted her beside me.'

'You did the right thing,' I told him gently. 'If you had to get out from something toxic, so did she.'

'And now I've lost her,' he said, tears starting to fall again.

'Did you lose her soon after you got here?' I asked, breaking one of my own rules, but keen to know if there was an injured dog out there.

'God no, no, not at all,' Tom told me, shaking his head. 'We've been here a while, you know how it is. You think you'll make a new life, do great things, then everything starts to go downhill and before you know it, you're trying to sleep in a shop doorway without someone spitting on you, trying to survive day to day without someone saying you're scum. I can never understand what makes people treat us like they do, I just want to be left in peace, yet that seems to annoy a lot of people. All I had was Poppy and she never left my side for a second. Until she had no choice.

'There's something else you don't know about me, Michelle – I'm asthmatic. I've had it bad ever since I was a little boy, and I've made some awful choices in my life that can't be excused, but what happened to Poppy was down to that.'

I knew a lot of street people who had severe medical conditions. Many of them had mental health issues, but there were also those with Parkinson's, MS, and a host of other problems. The streets were even harder for them because of the additional needs their illnesses presented. Billy and Doris had been my first intense experience with the problems homeless diabetics faced, and I had met many more since then. They'd had a wonderful outcome, which was the exception rather than the rule, and it sounded as if Tom had really struggled with his health.

'I could never really predict when I would have an attack, and I've had a few since coming here, but a couple of weeks ago was the worst ever. I can't even remember it – I've got most of this from other people.'

With no inhaler, no support, Tom told me of the night when he had collapsed in the street. Someone had seen it happen and thankfully called the police, although there wouldn't have necessarily been any recognition at that point that the collapse was due to asthma – drink or drugs would be assumed, I guess. When the paramedics came, they had something else to deal with.

Poppy.

Like all street dogs, she adored her owner and nothing – absolutely nothing – would make her leave Tom's side. As he lay on the pavement in the middle of a busy London thoroughfare, the paramedics were faced with the dilemma of a hugely protective Staffie who simply would not move from her place. Unfortunately, she had decided that her place was right on top of Tom's chest. They couldn't risk moving her – this was a completely unknown dog and, for all they knew, she could have attacked if they tried to shift her. They could coax, they could try and encourage her, but Poppy wouldn't shift. In the end, they had no option but to call the police.

When the police got there, Tom was still unresponsive and Poppy was still on top of him. The paramedics were getting worried and really needed to access Tom to see what they could do to help him. When the police dog unit arrived, they used their expertise and experience to persuade Poppy to leave her beloved owner for a moment, but she was so distressed at the sight of the paramedics treating him that the police had no option but to muzzle Poppy for their own safety.

'She wouldn't hurt a fly,' Tom told me, tears streaming down his face, 'but I couldn't tell them that could I? I was lying there, like an idiot, while they took my dog away.'

'You weren't being an idiot!' I assured him. 'You were ill, you didn't even know what was going on. If you'd been able to do anything, it would have been different, but you couldn't, which means we just have to look at what can be done now. Wherever she is – will they not release Poppy to you?'

'That's just it, Michelle,' his voice wavered, 'I don't *know* where she is. They took her from me, but no one will say where she is. If I don't get my Poppy back . . . well, there's nothing for me, there's no point to anything. I've been breaking my heart for three months and I still don't have my dog. Every day, every night, I ask every single person I meet, have you seen my dog, have you seen my Poppy? No one knows where she is. I've been wandering the streets, night and day, for three months now.'

The man was a wreck. Even allowing for him being homeless, he seemed shattered, gaunt and broken, and I honestly didn't think he would survive much longer if this went on.

'Do you want to see a picture of her?' he asked.

'Of course!' I cried.

He pulled out a tattered photo from his pocket that had obviously been taken in better times. He himself looked healthy and clean, with his arms around the most stunning Staffie I had ever laid eyes on.

'Oh Tom, what a dog!' I exclaimed.

Poppy was a dark brindle colour with flecks of white across her body, jagged streaks like Harry Potter's scar criss-crossed her coat, and suggested a magical creature to me as I felt an instant bond. She had deep, dark eyes and her head was slightly tilted back as she tried to snuggle into Tom behind her. She just oozed happiness.

'I can't do anything without her,' Tom wept. 'I can't sleep, I'm barely eating the scraps that people give me. I'm panicking when I think where she might be. What if she's had an accident? What if she's with someone who doesn't care about her? Nothing's right without Poppy. If I have her, I can get through, but if she isn't here, what's the point? I was told you could help me. I was told you are an angel. Please, Michelle, can you find my dog?'

'I'll have a damned good try,' I asserted. 'Right – tell me everything.'

Tom didn't have many details really, given that he had collapsed. All he knew was the street where it had all happened, the hospital he had been taken to, and that, no matter how many people he asked, no one could say where Poppy was. He was now in a hostel – which didn't take dogs – but he spent very little time there as he was always looking for her. He tried every time of night and day, thinking that he'd have more chance first thing in the morning, then changing his mind and feeling that the middle of the night might be more productive. He was dead on his feet. This couldn't go on.

'I'm not having this,' I told him. 'You did nothing wrong and she'll be heartbroken at the loss of you. I know a few places to try. Leave it with me and meet me here again tomorrow night at seven o'clock.'

'You're an angel, an angel on Earth,' he began, before I interrupted him to say that might be a bit premature, and he should really wait to see if I could do anything! However, I was on a mission. As I left the park, I looked back to see Tom slumped on the bench, a broken man with nothing ahead of him but a night without his beloved dog. Loneliness and grief had obviously been his companions from the moment he realised Poppy was gone, and I dreaded to think what would happen if I didn't reunite the pair of them.

I drove home and hugged all of my fur babies even closer that night. They were all so precious to me and I couldn't even imagine the pain I would feel if I lost any of them. This was the reality of it. All of us who love animals would do anything for them, no matter whether we have a comfortable bed at night or a damp sleeping bag caked with filth that we carry around from place to place. The thought of Tom crying himself to sleep in one of those sleeping bags without Poppy curled up inside it with him was a horrible thought, and I just hoped he could be strong enough to hold on while I did everything in my power to find her.

'I'd like to meet the person who would try to take you away from me,' I said to all of my babies as they looked up at me with big eyes. 'They'd regret it, I'll tell you that.' They all followed me to the kitchen where I made a cup of tea then sat down with a notebook. I made a list of everyone I could think, every individual and organisation, every support group and outreach worker that I would contact the next morning. If any of them knew the slightest thing about Poppy, I'd get it from them – and I wouldn't rest until I'd tracked her down. There was no doubt about this. I couldn't fail. I had to find Poppy the street dog.

NINE

Looking for Poppy

I tossed and turned all night, listening to the rain and thinking about Tom. Had he even found shelter or was he still sitting on that park bench, grieving? The truth was, if he had tried to stay in the park, he'd probably have been moved on, but I would bet my last penny that he had stayed there until the last possible moment, paralysed by grief. And what about Poppy? What if she was wandering the streets, looking for him, or, God forbid, what if she'd had an accident? The thought that she could be lying injured somewhere, or shivering cold, wet and alone, made my heart ache.

'Snap yourself out of it, Michelle,' I told myself in the dark. 'If that dog can be found, you'll find her. Tom needs you – and so does Poppy.'

I could only wish that meeting me had given Tom a glimmer of hope, and that he trusted in me to bring his beloved dog home. In my quest to find Poppy, I would be like the proverbial dog with a bone, which seemed appropriate, and I wouldn't rest until I had some information. It was true that, by this stage, the work with the homeless had taken over my life. Sometimes I did worry that there was a negative impact on my own family life, my friends and animals, but I did what I could. The kids knew how much this mattered to me and they were much older by now, with their own lives. My friends were supportive, though many of them didn't really understand what my street work entailed. My dogs and cats had everything they could ever have needed, and I made sure dog walkers came in every day, plus they got showered with cuddles and affection when I was there to such an extent that they probably needed to sleep it off every day!

I tossed and turned, but in the end, I decided there was no point staying in bed. Sleep wasn't going to be my friend that night. My mind was going at about a hundred miles an hour, which meant I was just as well getting up and preparing for the day ahead. I had a quick shower, dressed, fed the dogs, and went back to my list. A few more names had popped into my head in the early hours of the morning, so I added those and racked my brains while I took my own pups out for an early morning walk.

As much as I adored all of the street dogs I was now lucky enough to know, my own fur babies still gave me more joy than I ever thought possible, and every night when I got in, I hugged them that much tighter, thinking how lucky we all were to be able to curl up together on the warm sofa or bed.

By the time we got back from our walk, I was pretty sure that I had an exhaustive list and all I could do now was drink more tea and wait for the clock to hurry up.

As soon as it hit 9 a.m., I began.

'Right, Michelle,' I told myself as I got my phone from the charger and sat down at the kitchen table. 'You can do this. You can annoy people when you want to, you can pester them to get what you want, but, today, it's all about Poppy so make sure you get as many of them on your side as possible. We need an army out there looking for her just in case she is back on the streets. And if no one does help, well then . . . you'll just have to raise all hell, won't you?'

I called everyone I could think of and much of the information I received confirmed what Tom had said, along with some new pieces of the jigsaw to slot into place and help build a bigger picture of what had happened.

Tom had arrived in hospital and, as soon as he was able to, discharged himself to go and find Poppy. Little did he know that the police were already on their way to the hospital to let him know that Poppy was safe in holding kennels.

It was agonising to know how easily this whole situation could have been averted, because of course, when the police arrived, Tom had already left the hospital, which meant that they had no way of tracing him, and sadly, Tom didn't know how to go about finding out what had happened to Poppy.

It had been three months and Tom had been searching all the time, walking the streets day after day, trying to find his beloved dog. I knew that it was crucial for me to speak to Tom's caseworker, Emma. Luckily I knew a lot of the people working in the area by now, and before long, I was able to track her down.

'All he wants is his dog,' I told Emma. 'All he wants is Poppy.'

'I've tried, Michelle, I really have. I went to the police myself and logged a report, saying that he was out of hospital accommodation and that his health was on the mend, but they never looked into it. I've hit dead ends everywhere I've gone. I know that Tom is heartbroken, but what else is there to do? Poppy just seems to have disappeared.' Emma seemed very genuine and I believed that she had done her best – but I needed more.

I was well aware of how the system worked by this point and I was sure that she was still with the police. Before I called them, I sent an email to say I was trying to find a dog named Poppy who had been taken by the Dog Unit and that I would be phoning later, so could they please get some information ready in advance for me?

Someone must know something.

That was the thought that kept me going after many hours on hold and searching through contact names and numbers. There were so many rescue groups out there, all of them with a social media presence, and that gave me the idea to scroll through all the Facebook and Twitter and Instagram feeds. Tom had shown me that picture of Poppy, and the image of that dog was burned in my eyes. I would definitely recognise her if I saw her, I was sure I would. If there was any chance at all that she had been taken by a group and was up for foster or adoption, I would know it was her.

I set myself up for the rest of the morning, Bailey lying on my feet. I gave him a quick scratch, made what felt like my hundredth cup of tea, rubbed my eyes and got stuck in. I got lucky very quickly.

There she was!

There was Poppy!

On the page of a rescue centre I knew quite well, there was a very disparaging post about Tom. It was demeaning and completely false, saying that he was a druggie and that he had lost ownership of poor Poppy. The comments underneath were vile, an outpouring of hatred from people who knew nothing about the reality of life on the street and most certainly didn't know Tom's real situation. The rescue centre wrote that she was being transferred to them in two days from the police as her owner couldn't be bothered.

I was absolutely furious. That poor man had nothing to live for, was desperate for his girl to come back to him, and yet these people thought they could spread lies and encourage hatred of Tom without any consequences. *Not on my watch,* I thought, *not on my watch.*

I instantly called the guy who ran the rescue page and struggled to contain my rage as I spoke.

'What gives you the right to say these things?' I ranted, once I'd told him what the truth was. 'You're whipping up hatred and you're stopping a dog being reunited with an owner who loves her to bits!'

'You're the one who's wrong,' he told me. 'You've fallen for a pile of lies.'

'I most certainly have not – none of this is true, I don't know where you got it from as it's a complete fairy tale.'

He was fuming, I could tell that. 'I got it from the police, so take it up with them. Call them liars if you want.'

'I will!' I retorted. 'That dog is coming to me whether you like it or not.'

'No, she's not – whether *you* like it or not, she's coming here, and we'll find her a proper home. I have an interest in her, so she'll be mine in a couple of days.'

I might have let fly with a few choice words at that point and made it very clear – again – that I was the one who would get Poppy, not him. I'm afraid that, where animals are concerned, I find it hard not to speak my mind.

'There's nothing you can do. If you think I'm giving a dog to an unfit owner, you can think again.' With that, he hung up on me.

I called the police immediately, not waiting for them to reply to my email, just hoping that I was going to get to them quickly enough. I was in luck. I told them Tom's real story and they asked if they could speak to him, just to confirm it all. To my dismay, they said that it was unlikely that they could release her to him, knowing what his situation was and knowing that he was in accommodation where he wouldn't be allowed to keep her.

Tom! I hadn't told him that Poppy had been located! Everything had happened so fast, I'd barely had time to think. I jumped in my car and rushed to the little garden square where I had told him we could always meet. To my relief, I caught sight of him sitting there, but he was off the bench and running towards me as soon as he saw me walk in.

'Have you found her? Have you found my Poppy?' he asked, breathlessly.

'Yes, yes I have! But Tom . . .' I tried to calm him, but it was useless.

'Michelle, Michelle, Michelle!' he was crying. 'You're an angel, you know that? An angel. How did you do it? Where is she? Is she in your car?'

'Tom, listen to me, try and listen, OK?' He was holding my hands and nodding vigorously, but I knew that his mind was running away with him. 'I don't have her. I know where she is. She's safe. Do you understand all of that?'

He nodded some more. 'But is she in your car, Michelle?'

'Let's go sit down and take a deep breath.'

Shakily, he followed me back to the bench as I explained that the next stage would be for him to talk to the police.

'Then I can get her?' he asked breathlessly, his eyes wide.

'No, then we talk about what comes after that.'

I was so relieved to know that Poppy was safe, but I couldn't imagine how devastated Tom would be if he couldn't get his beloved girl back, and I didn't want to give him any false hope.

I called the number of the police officer I'd spoken to earlier. I confirmed who I was, and explained about Tom, before handing the phone over. I don't think I've ever been as tense as I was on that park bench, listening to Tom repeat himself over and over. He was getting more and more distressed in his desperation to get Poppy back, but I was concerned that he wasn't coming across particularly well, so I asked him if I could chat to them instead.

I was right. The officer asked if Tom would have any support in caring for Poppy if they were to release her. The phone was on loudspeaker and, on hearing the police officer's words, Tom got even more agitated. He tried to grab the phone from me, shouting, 'Give her to Michelle, give her to Michelle! Please just let me see my girl again.'

It took about ten minutes of back and forth with the officer, but to my relief, in the end, he agreed. If Tom wanted Poppy to be released to me, that would be fine with them. The police would deliver her to the dog unit at my local station where I could pick her up. It was more than we could have hoped for, and, leaving Tom with a broad smile on his face, I went home to try and pass the time until she had been transferred and I would be able to collect her. I couldn't settle for a minute, pacing the kitchen as I waited for that call. I knew that once the wheels were in motion, I would be able to reunite Tom and Poppy, which would be the most magical thing. I wasn't really allowing my brain to rush ahead to what would happen after that, though. Tom still needed help and Poppy still wouldn't be allowed into accommodation with him. I'd have to try and get her into foster care for a little while if I could, but I decided that I'd cross that bridge when I came to it.

When I got there, the police officer said he would take me out to their kennels.

'She's a lovely dog,' he told me, 'we haven't had any bother with her, but I have to say – she looks like her heart is breaking.'

It wasn't a warm, cosy environment for any dog. The kennels were very basic, with metal mesh doors and a stench of chemical cleaner in the air.

The police officer walked me over and unlocked the door.

'Can you just leave it closed rather than open at the moment, please?' I asked. 'I want this to be on her terms after all she's been through.'

'Sure, just let me know if you need anything. I'm glad she's got someone – I hate to see a dog like that, as if she's just given up.'

And there she was. There was Poppy.

She was just sitting there, in a corner, so bewildered and vacant. Street dogs pine for their owners when they are separated from them, and there wouldn't be a single person in the world who could have denied that this dog was in emotional pain if they had witnessed how she was acting. I was a little worried that she wouldn't be drawn to me because street dogs often like men more, given that's who they see most often, so I took it easy. This was my first real-life encounter with her and I took in every single bit of her. She was very chunky, a dark brindle with white jaggy stripes.

'Hello there, gorgeous,' I said, quietly. 'You've given me quite the runaround, do you know that?' I laughed. 'Look at those eyes. There's a story in those, isn't there? Well, do you know what Poppy? You've got a much better chapter coming up.' She did look up at me then, ever so gingerly, as if she wasn't used to someone just rambling on, asking nothing of her. She really did have the most gorgeous eyes. From that first moment, it was as if she was staring into my soul. 'You are gorgeous but I would never have pegged you as a Poppy. You look like you should be called Bruce!'

How daft was that? I was trying to make a dog laugh! I sat outside the kennel, just chatting, letting her get used to the sound of my voice. I couldn't let myself think about all she'd been through or it would have set me off.

'Your dad has been looking for you for months – you have no idea how much he misses you, Poppy. Well, maybe you do because you certainly look as if you've been missing him too. You know what? I'm here to take you back to him. What do you think about that? You'd like that, wouldn't you, Poppy?' I rattled on, telling her I would help, telling her that everything was all right now, over and over again. I put my hand to the door as I spoke, leaving it there without trying to persuade her to do anything but take it at her pace, and, gradually, she inched towards me. I could hardly breathe for fear it would send her back into the corner again, but after ten minutes, Poppy began to wag her tail and she sniffed my hand cautiously.

I knew we'd be OK.

She listened to every word I said, then I opened the kennel door and waited for her to come out to me on her own terms. Poppy crept towards me, the nearer she was getting, the faster her tail was going. By the time she was at my side, there was a huge smile on my face.

'Listen, Poppy,' I said, 'my bum is getting really cold. Can we go?' I laughed as she cocked her head to the side, wagging her tail as if she was asking me what on earth I was waiting for!

I hooked her up to a lead and walked her to my car, and the officer who had seen me in waved us off. Poppy walked beside me as if it was the natural thing in the world, and my heart went out to this gorgeous creature, knowing how confusing the last few months must have been for her. I put her in the car and called Tom.

'I've got her!' I could hear him whooping on the other end. 'She's in the car, safe and sound, Tom – how brilliant is that?'

'It's the best news!' he replied. 'And I've got news for you too – I'm leaving the accommodation I was put in as they won't have Poppy in the hostel. I'm going back on the streets. I'd rather have her than anything else. I choose Poppy.'

'You're what?' I gasped, horrified. 'Wait there, I'm coming!'

I drove to Westminster with Poppy in the back, ranting to her all the time that we needed to get her dad to see sense about his health. We'd find a way, but he shouldn't be making any rash decisions. She watched me the whole time, cocking her head to the side as if she was taking in every word. I just hoped Tom would be as attentive. Finally, we made it into the city.

'Right – are you ready? We're going to see Dad now!' I parked up and saw Tom walking towards the car.

As soon as Poppy saw Tom through the window, her tail started going like a helicopter propeller. She barrelled through the door towards her beloved owner as if she couldn't move fast enough. I thought she'd take off, her tail was wagging so fast, and if a dog could smile, I would have sworn she was beaming. Watching the two of them was like two long-lost loves reuniting. Honestly, I'd never seen anything so intense in my life. He was crying, I was crying, and Poppy was so, so happy. I waited until it had all calmed down a bit before I finally had to bring up the difficult issue that was worrying me.

'It won't be good for you or her to go back on the streets, you know that.'

'She's been in kennels for too long, Michelle. You have done everything for me, for us, more than I could ever have hoped for, but I won't lose my dog.'

'I'm not suggesting you give her up, Tom, but there has to be a way to keep you and her safe.'

'I agree that there has to be a way,' Tom said, taking me by surprise. 'I've been thinking about it while I've been waiting for you. I *will* stay in the hostel, but only if you foster Poppy and I can see her regularly.'

Although I was taken aback by this, I also breathed a sigh of relief. I knew Poppy would be fine with me, and I didn't have foster care sorted out anyway. I would be going home with another dog, but, I reassured myself, it was only temporary, so we could make do for now. 'Yes, yes, that's fine!' I didn't even consider all the animals I had already. I knew if Poppy and Tom went back out on the streets, it would just begin another cycle of him getting ill and her being taken away again, and I couldn't bear that.

'You two take as much time as you like just now, then I'll keep her for tonight, is that OK? I'll type out an agreement to say that you are behind me keeping her for a bit, just to make sure we're doing it all properly, then meet you tomorrow to sign it.'

Tom nodded, but he was wrapped up in Poppy really.

'Tom,' I repeated. 'Tomorrow morning, OK? Outside your hostel, nine o'clock. Do you get that?' Homeless people are notoriously bad at recognising time or even days, so I knew it had to be soon, and I thought if I made it early in the morning, I'd have more chance of him actually being there. I knew they didn't get kicked out of their accommodation until 10 a.m., which mean that, as long as he hadn't disappeared for the day, I would catch him.

Tom and Poppy cuddled into each other for a while, but when they said goodbye, I was surprised that she seemed absolutely fine to leave with me. She trotted along beside me back to my car and we headed home.

To my surprise, introducing her to my lot was far easier than I'd anticipated. I'd never had a street dog before, and although I'd got to know the ones on the street well during the three and a half years I'd spent doing outreach work independently, I still had no idea what to expect from a dog who had been taken away from everything it had ever known.

I opened the door and shouted, 'Right you lot – you've got a new sister!' Poppy stood there, waiting, but they didn't even bother getting up! When any new animal comes through the door, it's as if they think, *Well, we all came in the same way, needing help, and that's what this one is after too, so why make a fuss?*

'Look at this, Pops,' I said to her, 'bone idle the lot of them – do you think you'll manage this luxury for a while?'

Her trusting eyes and wagging tail suggested, yes, she would give it a damn good shot!

When Poppy came into my life from that day, she settled in straight away with my other pets. To my relief, there were no scraps with Bailey and Milly, no hissing or fighting with Freddy, Lolly, Pickle and Betty. It was just one lovely big furry family.

The next morning, after another sleepless night – partly made worse by Poppy trying to get under the duvet with me – I got out of bed, showered and dished out breakfast to my menagerie. I'd typed up a basic agreement the night before, just to say that Tom was voluntarily signing Poppy over to me without undue duress. I picked the piece of paper up from the table at my door, said goodbye to all my fur babies, and put Poppy in the car. Her eyes couldn't have looked sadder if she'd tried.

'Oh no, what's wrong, Pops?' I asked. 'Everything will be fine, I promise. Your dad just needs to get back on his feet.' She kept looking behind her, kept giving me puppy dog eyes, and I realised that there was a high chance I was being played.

'Now, tell me this, Poppy – is there any chance at all that you might feel a bit happier if you sat in the front seat?' I swear that dog understood every word I said. I opened the passenger door and she careered out of the boot straight into it. Driving into London, she looked pleased as Punch, as if she had found the throne she had always wanted! I'd have to watch out for this one; she had me wrapped round her finger already.

I walked, with Poppy, to the hostel where Tom was staying. Completely shocked, I saw him already waiting outside.

'You're up bright and early,' I laughed. I was so pleased to see him looking happy as I'd worried he might have changed his mind and be planning to go back on the streets.

'You know, this just feels right, Michelle,' he told me. 'Right for all of us.' We went for coffee together, he read the form, and then it was time for us all to move on to the next stage of our lives.

'I can't thank you enough for this,' he told me. 'She's a very lucky lady to have found you – we both are.'

Tom signed Poppy over to me that morning and I became her mum on 19 November 2015. I feel that if this was a Hollywood film, something would happen now. There would be dramatic music, or fireworks exploding, because this, *this,* was when everything changed.

It would be a learning process, living with her. Even though I'd lived with a lot of animals in the past, none of them were quite like Poppy. She had a very different history to Bailey and Milly. She wasn't bothered by either of them, but she was very possessive of me away from the house. If she thought another dog was heading for me, she'd bark and want to keep them away. I knew that, with encouragement and reassurance, she'd calm down.

For the first month she did struggle with things I never would have thought of, like adjusting to having central heating – she'd never had a regular source of heat, so didn't know that she could lie by the radiators if she was cold. She would shiver on the floor, not even lying on blankets for a while. Milly and Bailey loved their comfort though, which made her realise after a while that she could be a lot cosier. I had to introduce our noises bit by bit, things like my hairdryer, the TV or vacuum cleaner. Although she would have been around all of those noises before Tom left for the streets, it was as if she had been reprogrammed by street life and it did take her a while to stop cowering from them or running to another room, even though she wouldn't have flinched from a siren going off full blast. The thing with street dogs is that they never rest and they're never away from their owners. Poppy displayed that same behaviour even when she was indoors – she'd follow me to the loo, she wouldn't leave my side when I was having a bath and she'd sleep right next to me at night. She was a bit jealous of the others, but never in a mean or nasty way. If Milly or Bailey came to me, Poppy would jump on the sofa first to stake her claim, and I'd find myself sandwiched between all the dogs at once!

Every weekend, we would meet Tom in the Strand. Sometimes he would take her for a walk on his own while I did outreach work, sometimes we'd all go together. My view was, I was supporting Poppy in order to support Tom and it was working so far. She was such a loyal dog, but I guess her loyalty was being split now. It had been such a change in her life and she did enjoy her walks with Tom, but I was starting to see how much she enjoyed being an indoor dog too. She still loved Tom to bits and he was obviously finding it hard being separated from her, but what did the future hold, I wondered? I knew that, no matter what happened, if I needed to, I would keep Poppy forever, safe and loved. To my relief, Tom's health was much better now he was being supported and off the streets. Could it last? Would this current relationship last forever? I had no idea – it would be Poppy who decided.

TEN

The Longest Walk

One day, after about two months, she refused to go for a walk with Tom. It was as simple and as awful as that. It was like she had brakes in her paws; she dug herself into the ground, and wouldn't budge when Tom went to take her, but when I took the lead, she walked. I wasn't doing anything to make that happen, but she was clearly getting used to comfort and routine, and associating that with me, not Tom.

I could see the pain in Tom's face as he looked down at his beloved dog, the creature who had been his companion through the long cold nights and the endless days spent wandering the streets, and who now no longer wanted to go with him.

'It's time for me to say goodbye, isn't it?' said Tom, tears running down his face.

'No! She's just having a day!' Even though it was plain to see, I was trying to deny what was happening. Poppy was making a choice – and that choice was to stay with me, not go with her dad.

Pain was etched on Tom's face. 'It's obvious she wants you, Michelle. I can't give her the life you can. She deserves the best, she deserves everything you can provide for her. I want her to have a warm, soft bed, I want her to always know where her next meal is coming from – I want her to be with you. It's time isn't it, girl? It's time for you to go to your mum forever, Poppy.'

My heart broke at the sight of this huge man, reduced to tears once more for the furry creature he loved so dearly.

'No, Tom, no – this is something we can work through. You're just being stroppy aren't you, Pops?' I said to her, trying to coax her along, but the truth was, she was being anything but stroppy. She was calm, as if she had made a decision. And that was what Tom was doing too. They were together in this, just as they had been together in so many other things that I could only begin to imagine. I adored Poppy, but deep down, I realised that I had been waiting for some sign that she and Tom would be together. Maybe that he would pull himself together, find himself in a more stable position and get to a place where he could keep her and give her the life they both deserved. Seeing the two of them together now, it was starting to dawn on me that that might never happen, and deep down, I think Tom knew that too.

As much as he loved his dog, there were traumas and pain in his past that I would never know of, and because of this, it was always going to be difficult for Tom to live a normal life. He would be in a hostel, and that was the best we could all hope for. Meanwhile, the beautiful Poppy could be somewhere else, somewhere safe – even if that meant the hardest goodbye.

'Michelle – you have been a fairy godmother to both of us, but I need you to do one more thing. I don't want Poppy to be with anyone else. Will you be her owner?' Tom wept.

It was heartbreaking to see him in so much pain, but I knew I had to be strong for all of us.

'I would never, *never*, let anyone else take her,' I told him firmly, meaning every word. 'This dog has become one of my own, but Tom . . . this is something much bigger.' I tried to keep my voice steady, but the lump in my throat was getting bigger with every word I spoke.

'I want you to have her. I want you to be her owner,' he interrupted. 'This will be the last time I see Poppy.' As he said those words, Poppy moved closer to me and sat down at my side, perfectly calm as if she understood exactly what was happening. Tom bent down, gave her a kiss and one final pat before waving at me sadly and walking away, leaving behind the one creature he had loved above all others.

It was awful.

I felt responsible for breaking his heart. I'd only been fostering her; I'd had no plan to keep Poppy and I never would have wanted to break the precious bond between her and Tom. I knew how much they had needed each other, but I also knew that Poppy was the most important one in all of this. She had made her choice clear, and as much as I wanted to be able to fix things for Tom, I knew that some things were beyond my control.

Poppy was mine now, forever. Even in the short time I'd been caring for her, I'd grown to love her with a fierceness unlike any I'd known, and yet seeing the pain in Tom's eyes as he said goodbye made me want to sob.

I couldn't do any more that day; I felt absolutely drained, so Poppy and I went back home. The road back to my car was the longest walk I could have imagined.

'Looks like she's here for good,' I told Bailey as he nuzzled into me on my return. 'Looks like you have a new sister.'

As the day turned into night, I couldn't help but worry about Tom. What was he doing? How was he dealing with this? Was he walking the streets, was he back in the hostel? Was he drinking? Had he given up completely and would he end up back on the streets?

I didn't think I could do it after all. I rang the mobile I had given him, but it went straight to voicemail.

Tom – let's try again next week.

I left it an hour and tried again.

Tom, let me know you have picked this up – I think we should meet next week as usual. Poppy was just having a funny day – it'll be fine.

No reply.

All that night and the next day, I left the same message, over and over again. He never replied. He knew it was time to say goodbye, even if it was taking me longer to accept it.

Poppy was mine now and our relationship grew even deeper. She was officially part of the family and I loved her dearly, but I always thought of Tom. In my mind, I kept a window open. If he came back in the next three months, the next six months, the next year, we could go back. He might phone me; he might want to try again. I was living on thin hope – he never got in touch again.

Luckily, Poppy was a delight. That dog loved me to bits and I felt the same love for her. She just seemed so grateful for her new life. It was hard to get her on balanced dog food as she was such a scavenger – I guess she'd learned that on the streets, out of necessity, but we got there in the end. Not before a few hairy moments though. I remember it was coming up to Christmas again, and there was a box of mince pies on my kitchen worktop one day. I didn't think anything of it as I called out goodbye to the dogs. But when I came home, the box was torn open on the floor, and all the mince pies were gone.

Poppy was lying on the floor, her breathing was ragged and she hadn't even jumped up to see me when I got in, never mind be waiting at the door for me.

'Poppy!' I exclaimed. 'Oh God – have you eaten all of those?' It was pretty clear she had and I knew I had no time to waste. I admit I thought, *She's going to die*. I've never rushed to an emergency vet quicker in my life!

'Right, right, right,' I said more to myself than her. 'Car, vet, now!' She couldn't move so I bent down and lifted her up – not easily as she was a very sturdy girl – moving as quickly as I could to the door. I kicked it open and put Poppy in the boot when it opened automatically with my key. I ran back, shouted goodbye to the others, and closed the house door. I knew Poppy wouldn't be happy not to be in her preferred position of the front seat, but needs must!

I ran into the vets with her in my arms again.

'She's eaten a whole box of mince pies!' I yelled at the bewildered reception staff. 'Quick! Someone needs to make her vomit!' Hearing all the commotion, a vet came out and was as quick as lightning. Poppy was given charcoal injections to make her sick and, thankfully, it all came up really quickly. The vet told me that any longer in her stomach and she would have been gone. It cost me £600 but I was the one apologising to her all the way home!

'I'm sorry Poppy, I'm so sorry,' I wailed as I drove us home, weak with relief that she would be OK. 'I should have put them away; I shouldn't have left such temptation!'

I always say that a male dog can smell a bitch from miles away, and that's about the same distance Poppy could sniff out something she shouldn't eat. She was such a food scavenger that I had to get her on a strict routine. With life on the streets, the type of diet and the times of food are so inconsistent that the dog learns to eat when the homeless person does, often eating the same food as them. There's no regulation, which meant I had to impose that. It was a new world to Poppy to have food regularly every morning and every evening.

I was opening her eyes to a new world. She enjoyed her walks in our local park a great deal but tended to stick to Bailey as a playmate and avoid the other dogs. This was connected to her time on the street where homeless dogs don't really interact with each other. I decided to take her to a behaviourist to see if she could be let off lead as that was something I wanted her to enjoy, but I was scared that she might run off. I shouldn't have worried; she never took her eyes off me. It was lovely to see her be a dog and to have the life she was entitled to, that all dogs should be entitled to. Now when Poppy was exhausted, it was because she'd been at the park, playing with Bailey. When she lay down, she didn't need to be on guard, apart from his overenthusiastic grooming of her! She always had food and water, she always had a sofa or bed to curl up on when she needed to relax. I felt that she'd been given the world, but she had given me so much as well. I felt protected and safe when she was there, she made me laugh and she was a constant reminder of the streets and why I needed to keep doing the work I loved.

One of the things I really want you to learn from Poppy is how wonderful these dogs are. Although she was the most special girl in the world, all of these street fur babies are perfect in their way too. How many dogs do you know who self-train? Think of how long it took you to make sure your Daisy Dachshund or Sally Spaniel would sit on command, stop at every kerbside to check until it was safe to cross, give you a paw without question so that you could check for any injury. Now, imagine what they would be like in the middle of Oxford Street on a Saturday afternoon, just expected to sit there quietly, or even manage a nap in the middle of all the hustle and bustle. It just wouldn't happen, would it? It's not that one type of dog is better than another, it's that they all have their own worlds and they learn what those worlds are. Street dogs are constantly assessing things, for their own sake as well as that of their owners – where are we? What's going on? Are we safe here? Do I need to stay alert or is it OK to close my eyes for a much-needed kip? Dogs adapt so quickly to their circumstances, which is what gave me such hope that she would settle into her new life with me as well as she had her life on the street.

The more I got to know Poppy, the more I came to realise that, no matter what she'd gone through in the years before she came to me, none of her past mattered to her anymore. She was so content in her new life, and all she really needed was to know that she was by my side. Whenever I spoke, she would look up at me, her head cocked, looking as though she knew what I was saying, as if my voice took her back to that first day together in the kennels when I'd freed her. If I went out, the kids would phone to say, 'Mum, Poppy hasn't moved from the front door since you left!' She would sit there for hours, just staring, not even napping – waiting for me to come back. The moment I stepped through the door, I would be met with a rush of doggie kisses and the most enthusiastic tail-wagging I'd ever seen!

To my delight, as well as being my loyal sidekick, Poppy also loved Bailey and seemed to really connect to his amazing soul, his beautiful spirit. Bailey was such a gentle creature who immediately accepted his new sister, and before long, they were like conjoined twins! She blended in so well with our patchwork family, our menagerie of love. It was as if Bailey's aura drew her in and within days, they would sleep together, curled up tight around one another, looking utterly contented. They would play together when we were out on walks, and he would even wash her.

However, the first days and weeks were a learning process for both of us. Street dogs don't usually get on with other dogs, they're territorial, but Poppy was fine all in all. It was all so quick her coming into my home. She taught me a lot about Staffies. About the love they give and the security they provide. I could see why they used to be called nanny dogs. Sadly, Staffies are a very misun-derstood breed. They are the dogs most likely to end up in shelters and they are the ones who take longest to find new homes. They are overbred and often treated appallingly. The misconceptions about them make my blood boil, especially the belief a lot of people have that they can 'turn' at any moment. Any dog can do that if treated badly or threatened. You should always be careful mixing dogs and children, and make sure that little ones respect animals, never pushing them or pulling their tails, never encroaching on their space or messing about near their food. Media coverage tends to encourage this idea that they are a monster breed, but they have never seemed that way to me. Give a dog love and you'll get love back, that's what I say. They are such intelligent dogs and so easy to train, which is why you actually see so many not even on leads – they want to please and obedience is something that is inbred. Sadly, many people take advantage of this, which breaks my heart.

A lot of people also think they are a banned breed, which is a complete falsehood. They aren't any more destructive than any other dog who is ignored or neglected; they don't have 'locking' jaws or any of the other nonsense that is spouted. They are the most adorable creatures with the most beautiful faces *and* spirits.

It's true that Poppy would always have protected me if I was ever in danger but which dog wouldn't do that for their owner? I used to thank her for what she was teaching me – I can see now that Staffies look after you rather than the other way around and that she now thought I was the one who needed to be cared for and checked on. She felt she owned me, but not in a horrible way. My animals can sleep everywhere – beds, sofas, carpets, wooden floor – but Poppy was always lying on the sofa beside me, her head on my lap. I spoke to her all the time and it genuinely felt she was listening, understanding and taking in every word. Honestly, that was just what I needed. I worshipped all of my other dogs and cats, but there was something about Poppy that just got through to my core. It felt as though, all these years, she had been waiting for me and I had been waiting for her. Now that she was in my life, I couldn't imagine being without her.

It was eight years before Poppy found me, but it was a lifetime I had waited for her. There was a fate to being with Poppy that I truly believed was meant to be. That wasn't to minimise Tom's devotion to her at all, and of course I wondered how he was coping without her, worrying about what his life would be like without his beloved companion. I would never have done anything to separate Poppy from her owner, but the fact that she had chosen what was going to happen really did confirm my belief that dogs find you, choose you, and, ultimately, save you.

There was a lot of training to do – Poppy had to be 'de-streeted' and made into the dog she was born to be. It wasn't only the food that was a challenge – she even had to learn about water. Of course, there was always a fresh bowl of water there for her, but, to begin with, she still had the street attitude of only thinking she had access to it when her owner did. Poppy had to realise that she could help herself, not wait on me to give her permission to drink. I put water bowls everywhere to try to make her understand that it wasn't a rare commodity now, so that she could drink at all times. It was a lovely moment when I finally saw her go and take a long drink without any prompting from me, although for a while she lapped up too much at once, probably still feeling like she didn't know when she'd get it again.

At the start, I had been wary of Poppy's unpredictability if I let her off the lead. As time went on, I learned me that she was reliable and never showed any evidence of running away, but now I had flashes of wondering if she'd changed her mind and would run back to the streets. I bought her a special red collar and lead, with a plastic 'Poppy' key ring on it, and finally realised that she was going nowhere. Poppy was here for keeps. Before coming to me, she'd never worn a collar and lead before, but to my relief, she adapted really well.

If I'd known her and Tom before they were separated, I would have provided them with both on the streets, as I did with all the dogs and their owners that I knew, but because that hadn't happened, she had always just trotted along beside him, completely obedient and trustworthy. She took to everything so well and I couldn't have been more proud of her.

'You are the best girl in the world, aren't you?' I would croon to her. 'I think you and I were meant to be, Poppy, I really do. I wonder what you're going to bring into my life. You're here for a reason, I just know it.'

There wasn't a nasty bone in her; she loved affection and attention and gave it back tenfold.

'Are you under that blanket again?' I would laugh as she stuck her nose out and wriggled about in the bed, smiling at me as usual. I think she liked to be under blankets, probably from her days in a sleeping bag. I constantly worried that she'd suffocate though, always scared that something would happen to her. In reality, she was on top of things, and possessed a real street dog sense of what was safe and what wasn't to be attempted. She would stare at me with contentment when I was in the bath, leaning her head on the edge and there was nothing she liked better than for me to blow bubbles out to her. I swear I spent longer in the bath than ever before as she enjoyed it as much as I did! When she was groomed, I'd say to her, 'You are SO gorgeous, aren't you? You're my pretty, pretty Poppy girl.' The truth was, she was built like a tank! I'd thought that since the day I first saw her in the police kennel, and it wasn't as if she was going to change now, no matter how many times I took her to the groomer! She didn't even look like a Poppy as there was nothing feminine about her at all, but we used to laugh at that. Isn't it funny how we think that with our pets? That we're laughing together, that we're having a good old chat? I bet there isn't a person reading this story who doesn't feel the same thing, whether they have a dog or cat. There is just such a connection and the beautiful thing is that we can tell them all our worries, all our fears, knowing that they understand because they just love us unconditionally. It's a wonderful thing to have that fitting together that comes from person and fur baby, and I blessed the souls of every animal who came into my life and gave me such a gift. I watched the changes in Poppy and hoped that I was giving her a gift too. At first, she would sleep with her head down between her paws, then on her side when she felt a bit more settled, then on her back, legs up in the air and belly exposed when she felt safe and content.

'Happy now, are you?' I'd say, tickling her belly as she wriggled with delight. 'You've come home, haven't you, Poppy? You've finally come home and I couldn't be happier with that.'

It was true. She made me as content as I made her. However, I still had to do my outreach work, and while she sat at home watching the door for my return, I'd be back out on the streets, trying to help more dogs like her. Things weren't getting any better. Homeless people were still having to choose whether to access help without their dogs or stay on the streets with their canine best friends.

I never took Poppy with me on my outreach work as I was worried that it might traumatise her – I was afraid that she might think I was dumping her, putting her back into that life. Also, as I've mentioned, street dogs don't particularly like other dogs, which is why I was so surprised that she had cuddled into Bailey from the very start. I needed to keep her life consistent, which meant that I would do the outreach work on my own.

When I was on the streets, there was a constant refrain.

'Oh, you've got Tom's dog now, haven't you, Michelle?'

'Don't get ideas, I'm not taking any more!' I'd fire back instantly. It was funny that Tom had appeared to know so few people but many had heard that I had Poppy. I wondered what they thought of that and just hoped they knew what the circumstances were, that Tom had made the decision – well, Poppy had – and that it hadn't been something I had pushed for at all.

That time with Poppy opened my eyes. It was like having a dog from scratch. After so long living on the streets without any treatment or grooming, she needed lots of TLC, and I realised, more than ever, that street people needed free, accessible health and vet care for their dogs. These animals might not have been checked out by a vet for years, if ever. Every time I looked down at Poppy, curled up beside me on the sofa and thought of her life as a former street dog, the more I thought I had to fight for the rest of them who were still out there. Their owners were disadvantaged by not being able to access accommodation, but that didn't mean the dogs should be isolated from proper care and treatment.

I got my trusty notebook out and sat down at the kitchen table, just as I'd done when I pulled together that list for finding Poppy after she'd been taken from Tom. Naturally, she was beside me, her head on my lap, delighted that I was home.

'You've given me an idea, Poppy – and it's something that I might never have thought of without you. All of those dogs out there, all of them on the streets like you were, they can't be here in comfortable cosy houses, stealing blankets from their mum, but they need something. They need a *lot*. What can we do, Pops? What can we work out to make sure that they get even a bit of what you have?'

Poppy cocked her head, looking for all the world as if she was pondering my question! I gave her a scratch behind her ears and settled down to write.

My list soon grew.

Nutritious food

Water

Collar

Lead

Tags for the collar with my details so they could be linked back if they were found missing or injured

Toys

Treats

Blanket for winter

Cooling blanket for summer

Vet check-up

Flea treatment

Worm treatment

Tick treatment

Booster jabs

Spaying and neutering

Emergency care if they were hurt

Grooming

Training and advice

Microchip

That list only took a few minutes and I was sure that there were things I'd missed out. I was already providing some of it – food, treats, collars, leads and toys, for example, and had worked out that different blankets were needed for different times of the year – but there were huge things on that list too. I wasn't a vet and I wasn't a groomer. I wouldn't be able to directly help a dog if it was injured, and there were times when their owners didn't even tell me or notice a new condition in their dog, particularly if it had developed slowly or been going on for a while.

It was a daunting list already and possibly – probably – something that couldn't be achieved. Which meant I wanted to do it.

'Impossible?' I whispered to Poppy. 'Since when has that ever stopped me? Let's get started, girl. You've shown me what needs to be done – now let's go and change things.'

ELEVEN

And So It Begins

I started to put a basic plan together of what needed to be done to support the dogs living on the streets. I had the idea and a sense of what was needed, but I went back and forth, over and over my list, wondering how much of it could be done. What I needed was a place where I could set up regularly in Central London, where all of the street homeless with dogs would know where to find me, plus essentials such as an on-the-street vet, a groomer, helpers. Add to that the fact that they'd all have to be willing to work for free – not a big ask at all! This was a complex, large-scale undertaking I needed to pull together, not a simple one-off event.

I sighed at the thought of what might lay ahead of me if I was going to do this.

'What do you think, Pops, can we do it?' Scratching her behind the ear on her beautiful brindle coat always calmed me, and I kept telling myself that this was it – this was the reason she had come to me. 'You're not a normal dog, are you, Poppy? I've always known you're here for a reason, so let's get that reason underway.'

I knew that there was a large area at The Strand where food was given out at regular times, but that was for people. However, it was well-attended and word always spread to street newcomers that it was there, which gave me some hope. Services for dogs were sorely needed – given that I didn't know anyone else doing what I had planned for the street dogs, I wouldn't be stepping on any toes. I just needed to get everything in place and make sure everyone knew about it. I thought about everything I had access to as a dog owner and decided that these things were what I needed to be able to provide for those sleeping rough. If it was good enough for my Poppy, Bailey and Milly, why wouldn't it be what they deserved too? Over the next few months, Poppy was my inspiration. Every time she needed something, I'd think to myself, how do people out there get that? Dogs living on the streets didn't get what she did and I kept asking myself, why should that be the case for those other dogs? They should have everything, absolutely everything.

My wonderful groomer, Fiona, loved the idea of setting something up and agreed to help. I even managed to find a vet who would give his services for free. I advertised for volunteers and managed to get some start-up donations, both financial contributions and the things I would need for the dogs. I bought a second-hand car and decided that The Strand, where the food service was, would be a great spot for me to be at on a weekly basis. This was all organised in the space of just two months.

'Are we ready, Poppy?' I asked her. 'Have we thought of everything? I know it's just the start and I know that I won't realise everything we need until it's up and running, but we have to start somewhere.'

She looked at me with love as she always did, then cocked her head to the side, back and forward to get my attention.

'What are you trying to tell me, girl? Have I forgotten something? Food, treats, toys, vet, groomer . . . what's not on the list?'

Again, she was listening, again she was moving her head from side to side, as if prompting me to think a bit harder.

Suddenly it dawned on me.

'Poppy – you are such a clever dog! How could I have forgotten? We need a name!'

I wandered round the kitchen with Poppy at my heels, muttering *a name, a name*. It had to do what it said on the tin, it had to be something that reflected the fact that we were joining up the dots between what the people on the street needed, and what their dogs needed.

'That's it, Pops!' I squealed, skidding to a halt. Joining up the dots! **D**ogs **O**n **T**he **S**treet'. I was so happy. It was the perfect acronym and I'm sure Poppy thought so too, if the enthusiastic jumping and barking she was doing was anything to go by! Bailey and Milly came in to join us, and it was like our own little party. Everything was falling into place.

Now that I had the name, I could get a logo designed and then start printing leaflets, handing them out, raising awareness, and hope that we could get people to come along when we started. I set up social media groups and spread the word as far as I could. I talked to my dogs about it all the time, sharing with them my fears that no one would come, my worries that I had put too much energy into something that would be a failure. Poppy was my sounding board and, ridiculous as it might sound, she was the one I wanted approval from most of all. Everything I was doing was inspired by her and it was all for her. She certainly never complained or made me feel that I was doing the wrong thing, but who knows? Maybe she thought I was mad!

My first street-run dog station was on 12 March 2017, a beautiful sunny morning. I'll never forget that day. I packed everything up and off I went, kissing Poppy's gorgeous black nose before I left, for good luck, my stomach filled with butterflies. I felt such a huge sense of anticipation, but I also knew that homeless people often have no real concept of time so they might not even turn up.

When I arrived at our spot on The Strand, I quickly got going, setting up a green gazebo and a picnic table with all of the supplies on it. The vet met me there, with a vet nurse, a groomer, a trainer and a frontline volunteer. Everyone else seemed to share my nervous excitement, but I could tell they were just as keen as I was to get going. As I looked around at us all gathered there, I started to worry that there might be more of us than there would be clients! We were covered for every eventuality but, as the minutes ticked by, my worst fears were confirmed. No one arrived. We were all standing there, poised, waiting, but with nothing to do.

'It's the first one,' I assured all of the volunteers, trying to stay upbeat. 'People will have forgotten. They have a lot on their minds and don't really notice the time. Or maybe they lost the leaflet. Or maybe they didn't know what I was talking about or didn't think it applied to them.' I gave out a lot of excuses, trying to reassure everyone, but the truth was, I was terrified that this, my baby, had failed at the first hurdle. *What would I tell Poppy?*

I did feel a little dejected, until after an hour, at long last, I saw someone in the distance coming towards us. Fifi the Staffie! I knew her and her owner, Danny, from my outreach work. My first client! Fifi was checked by the vet and groomed, and was given flea and worm treatment. She got a coat and food, treats and a lead. She was the picture of health actually and must have been delighted at all of the attention that was showered on her. We were so excited as we crowded round her! All of that for one dog, but it was worth it. None of the dogs have leads on the streets, but that was one thing I wanted to change, and I was delighted when Danny was all for it too. I think he was overwhelmed at the reception they both got and that it was all free; we were just relieved to have seen our first dog. When Danny and Fifi were all done, we gave her a pink coat and off they went. Maybe I was imagining it, but Fifi seemed to have a new spring in her step, now that her gorgeous fur had been groomed and she had a new, smart jacket and collar to wear!

No sooner had Danny and Fifi turned the corner when I saw someone else I knew – Buddy, another Staffie, and her owner, Jimmy. This was fantastic! Buddy was given a red-check coat and all the same attention that Fifi had received – she too was perfectly healthy. It was a really happy atmosphere, and we ended up with four clients that day, more than I could have hoped for in that first desolate hour.

Another thing I provided was a dog tag with *I'm a DOTS dog* on it, my mobile number, and a specific reference number for each dog, so that I could link up to who it was – for example, number 2 for Buddy. I would link that number to the name of their owner, where they usually bedded down, and their caseworker's details, if they had one. If the dog got lost, I'd have all of the information. We microchipped any dog who needed it and I added my contact number to the database. I was scrupulous with all of the admin details that day and have been ever since. It's like a map of three lives – the dog, the owner and me. We are all connected and if anything goes wrong, the other services know who to contact immediately because of the dog tag and the microchip.

After that first session, I was elated – we all were. It was a privilege that anyone had turned up at all, and I decided there and then to go weekly, so that we would be established in the community and start to be a regular feature for people. I reached out to as many people as possible for donations to make sure I could continue, and lots of friends were very kind indeed. Some public donations also came in through social media. I was grateful for every penny.

By the time I got home, I was exhausted. Naturally, Poppy was waiting for me – whenever anyone was home with her, they would say that she always heard me and rushed to the door long before I would have thought the car was within hearing distance.

'Mummy's home and I've seen all your friends on the street!' I told her. 'Well, four of them, and that's enough for me today.' She loved me talking to her and I had plenty to say. I told her all about what we had done, who we had seen, what we had achieved, and she almost wagged her tail clean off! She was listening and wanted all of the talking I could possibly provide. Poppy stared at me all the time, but today she seemed to be taking an extra interest. 'What have you been doing?' I asked her, as always. After the mince pie debacle, I put cameras in every room, but she never did anything like that again and she seemed to have behaved herself that day. I used to be able to talk to her on my phone which played out of speakers when I was out, after Mince Pie Gate, but I hadn't had a chance to do that because I'd been so busy getting everything ready that day – it was just a relief that she seemed to have done nothing except lie in the hallway staring at the door, waiting for my return.

I chatted to Poppy for the rest of the evening, Bailey curled up at my feet, and I just felt so pleased that anyone had come along. I just wanted the word to spread now so that we could reach as many dogs as possible. I was already planning what we could do for the next one, buzzing on adrenaline. I went back out on my rounds for outreach work the next night, going to see all the usual places and people, and I also went out early on the Sunday morning to remind them all that the session was taking place.

To my delight, there were five clients at the second session, including Fifi and Buddy, who came for another visit. (In fact, Buddy and Fifi would be there every week, come rain or shine.) It was the same set-up, although this time quite a few members of the public came over and chatted to ask what we were doing. They seemed quite curious as to what was going on, and many people were shocked by the stories of the dogs and the way in which street people often had to choose between their best friends or accommodation.

From that first session in March 2017, it only took a few weeks before we were getting media attention. It was the newspapers that picked up on it to start with, with a mention here or there, and then before I knew it, by April we were being approached by BBC News and BBC London Live, picking up the story for TV. Word was spreading through the city and the country, and the homeless community was talking about it too, telling each other about all of this free care their dogs could have from Michelle.

More difficult cases began to appear quite quickly, often chronic conditions and those that needed further investigation or an operation. In order to handle these, we engaged with traditional vet practices for the complex situations that we couldn't provide treatment for on the day. One of the most important things for me was to get the dogs spayed and neutered, to prevent more dogs ending up as strays or living on the streets. As much as I believed in it though, spaying and neutering had to be the decision of the owners. I couldn't demand it, no matter how important I thought it was.

Within the first two months, we had seen every breed of dog and all sizes, some I hadn't even seen before in my outreach work. Those who were living on the streets with dogs did tend to know each other and they mostly had Staffies, Whippets, Staffie crosses, and American Bulldogs. The DOTS vet worked from nothing more than her backpack with the few provisions we had – we didn't even have sterile worktops. It was raw, pavement vet care.

The fact that all of our services were provided free of charge in an accessible setting, with no caseworker checks and no means-testing was hard for some of our clients to comprehend. They were so used to only getting help if there were strings attached, so I had to be blunt about it.

'Listen,' I would tell them, 'when have I ever let you down? When have I ever said one thing and done another? You guys know me by now. You've given me as much as I've ever given you – God, you're more my best friends than the people who actually *think* they're my best friends!'

They knew it was true. No strings, no frills. Just respect for them and love for their dogs.

Once we'd found our rhythm, and as news of the clinic spread through word of mouth and the media, we soon settled into a routine. The first year ran quite consistently and as time went on, the numbers only increased. We still provided the same service, at the same time, on the same day, with the same support. There was a huge demand for support on the veterinary side of things; I was providing a lot of the other stuff anyway, on a regular basis, not just Sundays, but vet support was something else. There were operations, investigations and consultations needed, and most importantly, consistency. In that first year, we were able to offer access to vet support twenty-four hours a day, seven days a week. That meant that we could get a call at any hour of the day or night, and for some reason it was during the night that we seemed to get most of the calls.

I guess it must have been panic. We all feel that way with our pets, don't we? Everything seems worse in the middle of the night, in the dark, when our minds imagine awful outcomes and fears seem bigger than they are in the cold light of day. It was understandable panic mode and we were the ones who were available. I was thankful that we could offer that service and that support.

I remember someone called Mark phoning me up at about 3 a.m., crying down the line in complete distress.

'Michelle! Michelle! You've got to help me,' he cried. 'My dog's winking, and she doesn't normally wink! Something's wrong, I just know it.'

'Mark, Mark, calm down,' I told him. 'This is about Clover, right?'

'Yes, yes, Clover's winking!'

I sighed deeply. 'Dogs wink, Mark. Dogs wink.'

'*She* doesn't!'

'I can assure you she does. Tell you what – if she does become ill, phone me tomorrow, OK?'

'You sure, Michelle?'

'Yes, yes, I'm sure. Winking's fine, it really is.'

I'd have a bit of a swear to myself but realised that even these minor things could get blown out of all proportion and now that there was help available, it was much easier to offload onto someone else. The good thing was, it meant they felt reassured and comforted by what I was doing.

After a handful of calls that jolted me and Poppy awake

in the early hours, I did have to have a chat with people to rein it in a little bit. It had to be made clear that the only way we could provide 24/7 support would be if they knew to only use it for emergencies, not for basic stuff that could wait until the next day.

Sundays were working really well, but during the week, I was still 'operational' as it were, and still seeing all the rough sleepers as much as ever. We had found a sort of halfway house to run alongside the emergency 24/7 line whereby the vet and I would work as a mobile outreach team, with me acting as a sort of triage filter to see what really needed more detailed assistance.

If DOTS had to take a dog in for an operation, the procedure would vary regarding when it could go back onto the streets. For basic neutering, we would wait until the anaesthetic had worn off during the day and then they would be fine – they recover remarkably quickly. However, if it was something more intense, then after the procedure, I'd get the owner and dog booked into somewhere like a Travelodge for a few days or however long it took for recovery. It all depended on vet advice. Basic things such as sedation or minor ops could often see the dog back the next day or having an overnight stay at the vet surgery, but with something more intense, we'd weigh up the situation with the owner and their stress of being away from the dog, hopefully giving them a bit of respite. Getting into hotel accommodation could be an odd thing because, although the owner could have a bath or shower, some food and a comfy bed, make sure the dog was OK, I never had an instance of someone begging me to make that a permanent option for them, or angling for an overnight stay if it wasn't needed. They knew the streets, and for many of them, that was their home.

What they didn't know was how to organise anything. I always arranged transport to the surgery or to the hotel as they wouldn't know in a million years how and where they needed to get to. I couldn't risk them being late for an appointment or getting lost – I knew I had to keep everything on schedule, especially if a dog needed an early-morning operation.

DOTS was getting more and more attention all the time, not just from rough sleepers but from members of the public too. Sometimes people would come to the Sunday session with bags of donations, trying to do some good but often missing the mark completely. People do try to be kind when they give us things, and I'm always so appreciative and am overwhelmed by the generosity of strangers. I have to admit that it would help so much more if people could just think a little more about the things that they are donating. Street dogs are very territorial, and can often be defensive around other dogs, so there is no way that I would make them use a second-hand coat or harness still covered in the previous dog's hairs. It would be like putting another dog on top. I often hear the saying *Beggars can't be choosers*, as if those on the streets should just fall over in gratitude at any scraps that get tossed their way, and I'm afraid that this does make me cross. Everyone deserves dignity, and no one ever knows whether they might one day end up in the very position they look down upon now.

I had to be quite firm about it after a while, when people turned up with a jumble of assorted odds and ends, and say, 'No, thank you,' and suggest other ways they could help.

It was all a learning process, that's for sure, but there was still a long way to go. Throughout that whirlwind first year, I tried to keep on top of everything, and Poppy was my saviour during that time. For every late-night call, every early-morning operation or last-minute drama, she was by my side to remind me why I was doing this work, and to help me remember the dogs at the heart of it. No matter how much I thought I knew, though, I don't think I would ever have been able to prepare myself for some of the things that were coming my way.

TWELVE

Lena

The streets are home to hundreds of men and their dogs, but there are a few women out there too. They are usually either very young or quite old. The young ones often fall into two categories – girls who have been brought up in care and are left to fend for themselves once they turn sixteen, or much older women who have been through a lifetime of addiction and trauma. However, there is a common thread which runs through the stories of women on the street though – they are generally victims of exploitation once they get there.

People often ask me how many people are sleeping rough, but I can never answer. It's partly because I only see the people I see, if that makes sense. I'm there with my agenda, which is to help dogs and their owners, without making them fill in forms or jump through hoops, but when it comes to homeless women, even if I spent years researching the numbers, I couldn't tell you how many there are. This is because they aren't even counted. Wales and Northern Ireland don't report the numbers of females on the streets, so there is no way of getting a UK figure. For a lot of survey results, there is a count made of people bedding down on a single night, but they generally exclude those who are wandering around, drunk or high. This way of counting works against women in another way – many of them refuse to sleep on the street as they won't risk getting into a sleeping bag and curling up for the night because it makes them even more vulnerable. They have to keep moving and can't risk staying in one place for too long, because, for all the abuse so many of the homeless community receive from some members of the public, women are subject to an even worse level of treatment, often seen as fair game by some of those same male members of the public. Homeless women of all ages are frequently offered money, food or a bed for the night, in exchange for sex.

One night, as I was walking through Westminster looking for anyone who might need help, I was quite surprised when a teenage girl approached me. Most of the people I worked with tended to be male, as women often stayed hidden.

'Hello,' she said, her steps falling into time with mine.

'Hello, I'm Michelle,' I replied.

'I know – everyone knows who you are. I'm Lena. Can I help you with the dogs?' she asked.

'Of course you can – do you have one?'

She shook her head sadly.

There was something about Lena that made me think the dogs could wait for a little while – I had all night, after all, and she looked as if she could do with a listening ear.

We popped into a late-night café, where I got her a cup of tea and a fry-up. She was a skinny little thing, and as I watched her from the other side of the table, I couldn't help but think of my own daughter. The very idea of her being exposed to life on the streets was unthinkable.

'You like dogs then, Lena?' I asked her.

Her face lit up. 'I love them. Never had one but, you know, maybe one day . . .' Her voice trailed off. 'Michelle, I know you help the dogs, and everyone says how kind you are, but do you help people too? People like me?'

'I help whoever I can,' I said. 'Do you need something?'

It was like taking down a flood defence. We sat in that café for an hour and Lena poured out her heart to me. She opened my eyes to so much of what was going on with homeless women, women who had been sold for sex, as she had. She told me of other girls who had been pimped after being found on the streets. Some of them had been trafficked to the UK, with London being a major hub for that, and some had been kicked out of home and exploited by men who look for lost souls in major train stations or travel centres such as King's Cross. The buildings which housed all of these girls were nothing more than squats really. Horrible, soulless places with filthy mattresses on the floor, where the women even had to ask permission to go to the bathroom. They would be punished for the slightest thing: not 'seeing' enough men that day, complaints by abusers that they didn't look like they were enjoying it, that they seemed upset by the appalling things that were being done to them. If the women were from abroad, their passports were confiscated by the traffickers so they would have no way of escaping – and, as they were here illegally and often spoke no English (apart from sex words they were taught), they had no idea of how to access help. Not that they would be allowed outside without someone accompanying them anyway.

Lena was in the category of those women who come down to London believing that it will be the start of a wonderful new life. She was one of those who had been taken into care after a horrific home life, and only planned to sleep rough for a few days until she got her bearings. She thought she'd walk into a job in a shop or café, get enough money to rent somewhere, and soon have the city at her feet. The reality couldn't have been further from the truth.

After sleeping rough for a few days, she was dirty and unpresentable. She wasn't sleeping as she was scared, and the little money she had with her was stolen by another girl who had pretended to be her friend. Lena thought it was this girl who tipped off a man called Robbie, who found Lena within only two weeks of her being in London. Robbie was a smooth talker – as they all are – clearly not homeless, but looking for attractive girls who were down on their luck to work in his bar. Lena was delighted. Robbie told her he'd be back the next day with more details, but before he left, he gave her some money to get a hot meal, and made her feel that finally she'd caught a break.

'He came back about three days later,' she continued, 'not the next day, so I'd been getting really worried. I thought he'd decided I wasn't what he was looking for, and who could blame him? I was a state by then, it had all gone downhill so quickly. By the time he did turn up, I was just so grateful . . . so grateful.'

Watching her speak, my heart broke for her. She was so young and vulnerable, and it was terrible to think of a man like that going out of his way to exploit her for his own gain.

Sadly, though, it's how scum like that work. These girls have nothing. Lena was already feeling lost and desperate. He had got her hopes up and I had no doubt that he had deliberately left her for longer so that his return would make her feel even more thankful to see him. Although there are outreach services looking out for young women on the streets, unfortunately they didn't find Lena in time – Robbie was much quicker than them, and probably much more experienced.

'When he came back, he was a bit more distracted,' Lena explained, chewing on her fingernails shyly, and barely able to meet my eye. 'He'd been really flattering to me before, told me that it was such a shame that someone as pretty as me was in this situation. He even said that the thought of his little sister ever being on the streets like me broke his heart, and that was why he wanted to help me. He only wanted to help himself though, didn't he, Michelle?'

What could I say? Of course he did, but there wasn't any point in making Lena feel any worse than she did. She went on to tell me that Robbie had said that there was a vacancy that she might be suitable for, though it had now changed from a bar to a club, and it had changed from an opportunity that was hers for the taking to something that she would have to prove she deserved.

As Lena spoke, I could see her eyes becoming more glassy, she was swaying from side to side, and even her love of dogs had disappeared under layers of self-loathing.

The club she had been promised didn't exist; instead, it was a brothel. She was taken by Robbie to one of those filthy rooms I'd heard about and told that he needed her to do him a favour. If she did this *one* favour, then he'd make sure she was OK. He'd get her a job and she'd be sorted. The one favour turned into a few which turned into a few more, and before she knew it, the only thing he was giving her were cheap takeaways and drugs. Any time she tried to complain, she'd be met by his fists and a reminder that the door was locked and he had done her a huge good turn by getting her off the streets.

'I don't even know how long I was there for,' she told me, her voice hollow.

I knew that disconnecting from what had happened was obviously the way she had learned to cope with the terrible things she'd experienced, but it was still so sad to see someone so young talk in such a detached way about the horrific things that had been done to her. The things she told me were so appalling that I can't even repeat them here.

'How did you get out?' I asked gently, not wanting to probe, but sensing that it was a relief for her to get the words out. Even though she was still only a very young girl, she had big dark rings under her eyes and she looked haggard, the drugs and abuse having taken their toll on her mind and her body.

'He kicked me out one day. It was odd – he didn't hit me or punch me, he just opened the door and told me to get lost. Well, he didn't say it quite as politely as that – he shouted and said I was no use to him as he'd been getting complaints and the streets were the best place for me.'

'Oh Lena,' I said, giving her a hug. 'You don't have a dog so you can get accommodation, you can get help.'

'What's the point?' she asked. 'Robbie was right. I'm no use to anyone.'

She was shaking, obviously withdrawing from whatever drug he had given her. Everyone I met on the streets knew I would never give them alcohol or cash, and to be fair to them, most never asked. In the time that I knew her though, Lena did try a few times. Each time, I refused.

'How do you think I would feel if I gave you a fiver and you bought something that killed you?' I asked. 'How could I live with myself?'

As much as I wanted to try to get her some support and a stable place to stay, she was fiercely independent and wary of the authorities, and was therefore really against the idea of getting help, despite the fact that Robbie was circling again, seemingly looking for another opportunity to brutally exploit her.

All I could do was be there for her when she wanted to talk, and support her as much as I could. Each time I saw her over the next few weeks, I had to let her return to the streets, possibly back into Robbie's clutches. I often found myself lying awake at night wondering what terrible situation she might have found herself in.

I felt pleased that at least she felt able to talk to me, and we got to know each other quite well. Even though she didn't have a dog, she loved all of the street dogs and relished getting cuddles from them whenever she could. I asked a few of the guys to look out for her, the ones who would never have taken advantage, and they managed to do that for a while by encouraging her to play with their dogs and take an interest in them. All the time though, I knew Robbie was never far away and there was only so much I could do to keep her safe. I gave her names and numbers, I told her of programmes that could help, but she was ground down and felt that she was worthless.

One day, I couldn't find Lena anywhere. Or the next day. Or the next. No one had heard from her, none of the other outreach teams, or the few women I did know on the streets, or the blokes whose dogs she had loved. She was just gone.

Of course, there was a part of me that hoped she had struck lucky, but I knew how unlikely that was. I felt devastated to think of a vulnerable young girl like that falling prey to Robbie again, or another person who would take advantage of her.

At the Sunday Strand session, I asked around again to see if anyone knew where she was. It was only at the very last moment, when one of the regulars said he'd seen 'that scumbag' with Lena, that my worst fears were confirmed. No one knew where she was.

He'd done the same as he had to begin with, I guess. Played the long game by ignoring her, then making her feel he was her only option and that she should be grateful for what he offered. I had no doubt that she was back being used for sex, in that horrible room, twenty-four hours a day, completely dependent on Robbie for drugs. I almost hoped she was completely out of it given what was being done to her.

It was about a month later that I was suddenly jolted awake by the sound of the phone ringing. It was past two in the morning. As the 24/7 mobile number wasn't being abused quite as much – no winking dogs anymore! – I was immediately worried that there was something seriously wrong, and my heart was in my throat as I answered.

'Michelle!' said the voice on the end of the line. 'It's Bob, Cato's dad.'

Cato was a gorgeous little white Whippet who had been on the streets with his owner long before I started as an outreach worker. He must have been quite old by now and my heart sank.

'Oh Bob, what's happened? Is it Cato?' I asked, worriedly.

'You'd better get here as quick as you can, Michelle. It's not Cato – it's that lass Lena. She's in some state and she won't talk to anyone but you.'

Bob told me where she was – a street near Soho, one of the areas that the rough sleepers were never keen on me visiting. I pulled on some trousers and a warm sweatshirt, said goodbye to the dogs (Poppy was already on guard at the door, sensing that I was heading out), and drove there as quickly as I could. The streets of London are never quiet, there is always noise and light and people wandering about, but as I got close to Soho, I could see police lights flashing and an ambulance parked. I raced to park the car, leaving it at an angle that would have guaranteed me a ticket or a towing during the day, and ran, too scared of what I was going to find to worry about traffic wardens.

As I rushed over to the scene, I could see that Lena was sitting on the pavement, covered in blood. She was wearing nothing but a skimpy lace nightdress, and she looked terrifyingly thin and vulnerable, surrounded by police officers, paramedics, Bob and Cato and even a couple of builders, for some reason, and she was sobbing her heart out.

When she saw me, she tried to get up but was obviously weakened by drugs and whatever had happened to her.

'What has happened?' I asked, as I reached the poor girl. All I wanted to do was to wrap her in a blanket and take her home as I'd have done one of my animals, but I could tell from her injuries and her thin frame that she needed far more serious help than I could ever give her.

At long last, I got the story from about eight different people. It turned out that Lena had jumped out of a third-floor window to escape the sexual torture she was being forced to endure. She had decided that she would rather kill herself than go through that torment for a moment longer. Thankfully, her fall had been broken by two builders who were working on replacing broken parts of the pavement at a quieter time when there were fewer pedestrians.

She was covered in cuts and bruises, some of which looked as if she'd had them for a while, whilst others were clearly fresh. It was obvious that she needed medical treatment, but she had refused to move or talk until someone called me. There were armed police trying to get into the building that was housing the brothel and Lena was completely traumatised.

I sat down beside her and tried to calm her down as best I could. At long last, to my relief, she agreed to go with the paramedics. She was taken to hospital with cuts and bruises, and, miraculously, only had a sprained ankle. Those builders had saved her life – but what sort of life was ahead of her?

I went home that night with a heavy heart and buried my face in Poppy's soft fur. For all the positive work we were doing, sometimes the realities of life on the streets were just so devastatingly harsh. As much as I wanted to save as many people as I could, I knew that there were situations that were far beyond my control or expertise.

Lena discharged herself after a couple of days. She needed a fix and hobbled straight back onto the streets to what she knew. I did what I could for Lena, trying to keep track of her and asking the guys to look out for her as much as possible, but apart from checking up on her and feeding her when I did see her, she wouldn't accept anything else from me, and wouldn't let me put her in touch with any other support.

She hated the other outreach teams as she said they patronised her and couldn't see past her drug addiction. She was certainly still managing to get a fix while rough sleeping, and I dreaded to think where she was getting the money from. The only time I really saw her smile was when she was with one of the street dogs, especially Cato, as Bob was looking out for her when he felt up to it.

I knew in my heart that Lena would never have been able to take care of a dog of her own. It was never an option. All I could hope was that she would experience a little brightness each day by hugging the others and their dogs, getting that contact.

I don't know what happened to Robbie or his horrible 'business'. Even if he did get shut down, even if he was prosecuted, there are plenty of other men like Robbie in London and far too many places where young women like Lena have their hopes and dreams taken from them.

I'm sorry to say that I don't know what happened to Lena. I'd love to give you a fairy-tale ending – to tell you that she went on to study to be a vet, that she helped out at the Sunday Strand sessions and was encouraged to do more with her life, that she rescued a puppy herself and found that it was her salvation, but none of that is true. She just disappeared, like so many do on the streets of London – sadly I have no idea where she is.

No one plans to become homeless; they don't have it as their life goal. It's just what can occur when things don't go as they should. Life can be cruel, things happen that we can't control, and sadly there's no easy answer or solution. People often say, *Why not call your family or friends?* Unfortunately, it's not as easy as that either. Homeless people feel shame and embarrassment, they have pride and they often feel they are protecting their loved ones from the reality of their situation. Things get worse and worse for them, and they dread the idea that their parents or siblings or spouses would see what they've become. Of course, homeless people aren't all the same, but these are common themes that I see over and over again in my line of work. There is no one route into homelessness, just the truth that it is far easier than any of us dare think to spiral from one bad decision or choice to another, into more and more things that go wrong.

Everyone has a story. Every homeless person I work with has been changed by living on the street – the only common thread that goes through the people I know is the dogs. Everyone can be changed by getting off the streets, but if they can't take their precious friend, this isn't even an option. Their dog is often their only companion, the only thing that gives them hope, a bit of love and affection, but Lena didn't even have that.

I wish I could have given her more. I wish that she could have used that instinct and trust she had for me – the same trust that made her force Bob to call me – because I know if she had, we could have run with it. I can't be an expert in everything – in fact, I sometimes feel that I'm an expert in nothing when it comes to the streets. Although I love and respect street people, and I will fight to my last breath to give them dignity, I do feel that it is by doing practical things for the dogs that I can make a difference. I couldn't have made Lena's life perfect, but I can look after dogs. I can get them food and vet care and blankets.

I can make sure that their owners always have me at the other end of the phone, be there day and night if there is a worry or a tragedy.

It's all I can do. After my time with Lena, I learnt that the issues for rough sleepers, especially women, are greater than anyone can imagine. There is a world of exploitation and horror out there, the likes of which ordinary people would struggle to comprehend. All I could do was keep chipping away at the little bit of that world I had been given access to. *Focus on the dogs, Michelle*, I told myself, *they're the ones you can help, they're the ones whose everyday lives you can change.* I needed to keep strong; I couldn't allow myself to wallow in stories like that of Lena. Poppy would keep me on the right road. She'd always made sure of that so far, and I didn't think she would let me down at any point soon. *Keep to the Poppy path, that's your guiding star*, I would say after a particularly rough time. Poppy – just focus on Poppy.

THIRTEEN

Come on, Poppy

By now, I had come to realise that I just 'got' the homeless. Like them, I felt I had nothing to lose. I'd been in situations in the past where I'd had my soul battered too; I'd been invisible for much of my life, seen people close their eyes to the things I was going through. I think that's why, even though I do have a few friends in my non-DOTS life, they don't seem as real almost as those on the streets. I am not the sort of person who welcomes people popping round or just turning up at my door; I much prefer my own, solitary company or that of animals. I'm scared to get close to people in case they cheat me or betray me, but dogs stay with you, they never go – they stay with you in spirit forever. With rough sleepers, there is an honesty to them that I appreciate so much. They're very genuine and that matters a great deal to me. I can be me, so I'm at my happiest around them, and this is just as well for me because it's difficult work.

I have seen everything you can imagine. When you're spending so much time working with homeless people, you experience it all – the complex backgrounds, the PTSD, the trauma and abuse. I absorbed that from the moment I began working on the streets and I don't – I can't – switch off when I go home. I've seen people die in front of me, I've struggled through identifying people with nothing but their dog's tag as a clue and I've even had to deal with someone becoming obsessed with me, with delusions that we were married.

People are wrong if they think the homeless lie and cheat and manipulate. Of course, there are good and bad just as there are in any group, but I keep going until they know I won't give up on them and they treat me well as a result. Their thoughts and fears change by the day, which means I have to respond to that. They will sit and cry with me and that is such an honour. I never promise anything though. If I say I'll do something, I'll do it, I don't need to promise.

After the first session in March 2017, the next few months into summer were a total whirlwind – I felt as though I hardly stopped for a moment. If you had asked me during that period to describe how I was feeling, the only word I could have used would have been *wow!* I couldn't really believe how far we had come in such a short time, but I felt immensely proud that, despite our rapid growth, we were still providing an exceptional level of service. However, it still wasn't the full extent of what I wanted to provide.

Despite our initial success, I couldn't stop my mind from racing ahead. Over and over again I found myself thinking, *If we have managed to do all this in the first few months, then what are we going to achieve in the future for these people?* There was no limit to what DOTS could do – we were flying.

In the early days, social media was vital to us. We started posting a lot, and people who wanted to help saw our wishlists and appreciated exactly what was needed. Our website was developed and we developed the DOTS brand, using orange everywhere because it was the colour of Poppy's collar, and ultimately she was the true inspiration behind all of this.

Every time I came back from a Sunday session or an outreach, there she would be, sitting at the front door where she'd been since I left, delighted to see me. I'd get a dog walker in if it was going to be a long day, and I'd check on the doggycam every now and again to make sure she was safe and wasn't getting up to anything naughty, but I'd stopped chatting to her while I was away, as I realised that hearing my voice when I wasn't actually at home would be confusing for her. To my relief, she seemed perfectly happy to just wait for me. I know she must have napped a bit, but every time I came home, she gave the impression that her eyes hadn't moved away from the door for even a moment. I'd come in and she'd be wagging her tail enthusiastically, barking with delight, having already heard the car, and we'd sit on the doorstep and have a cuddle as if we'd been apart for years. She was just so full of love and was never shy of showing it. It was the true highlight of every day, coming home to her beautiful, grinning face. I'd tell her all about my day, or night, and she'd listen to every word. It seemed to me that Poppy was never happier than when I was talking to her, her wise eyes fixed on mine as though she was taking it all in.

'I wonder what you'd say if you could answer me, Pops?' I would ask her. 'Am I doing the right thing? Am I missing something? What would your little friends like that I haven't thought of?' She'd just shove her nose into my leg or my arm, wherever she could snuggle, and smile. I was sure she was saying, *You're doing just fine, Mum, you're doing just fine.*

My house was my own precious little sanctuary. The dogs and the cats were all I needed when I got home after each trip into Central London, and they listened to my worries as no human ever did. To my delight, Poppy was adjusting to what must have seemed to her a new, luxurious way of life. She knew that she always had access to food and water, no matter what, that she could sleep in a comfy bed every night (mine!) and that she could even rely on Bailey to groom her at times. It was a complete turnaround for the street dog who had stolen my heart.

'You're liking your home comforts now, aren't you Pops?' I would laugh at her.

One Sunday, I had just got back from the usual Strand session and she was at the door waiting for me. 'Right, let me get the kettle on and then you and I will have a good old natter,' I told her. 'It was soooo busy today, and really hot as well. I saw lots of your friends but it's picking up every week and I bet you wouldn't know half of them. They probably wonder who Poppy is when everyone talks about you!'

We went through to the kitchen, I got a cuppa, and all of the dogs got a treat before I kicked my shoes off and flopped onto the sofa. 'Mummy will just have five minutes before she starts on the admin,' I said, yawning. The heat was really getting to me that day. August had hit hard and there was blazing sun almost constantly. I had given out unlimited bottles of water and cooling blankets at the van but I couldn't help feeling anxious that the street dogs would get too hot unless they got shade from the afternoon sun. Their little paws couldn't cope with the hot city pavements and I was really concerned about them all.

I lazily scratched Poppy's tummy and chest as she lolled on the floor beside me, hanging my arm off the sofa to give her a good old rub – when I stopped short.

'What's that, Poppy?' I asked her, trying to keep my voice bright. 'What's that on your chest?' It felt like a lump, but I told myself I must have been mistaken – I checked her all over for ticks, injuries, scratches, trying not to let my imagination run away with me. There was no denying it though. As I ran my hand over her chest again, I knew with a horrible sinking feeling that it definitely was a lump.

'Oh Poppy, what's the matter with you, darling?' I fretted, unable to stop my thoughts from spiralling. 'That's a lump for sure – we need to get you to the vet pronto.'

I couldn't sleep that night, frantic that there was something wrong with Poppy, and by the time I got her to the practice in the morning, I had a knot in my stomach that just wouldn't go away. To my relief, the vet working that morning was Brian. We knew each other well – in fact, I sometimes joked that I kept them in business with all the animals I took in! – and he was extremely reassuring. I had a few vets who I trusted, but this was the surgery that was closest to my home so seemed the best one to choose.

'I know it's worrying, Michelle, but Poppy's only eight. She has a great life with you now, she's healthy and more often than not, a lump is nothing to worry about. Most of them are completely benign and you've done the right thing getting her here as soon as you found it. Come on, Poppy,' he said to her kindly, 'let's get you looked at and put your mum's mind at rest.'

I held Poppy close as Brian drew some cells from the lump with a needle. To my relief, she was as good as gold while it went on, and lay there obediently until it was done.

'We'll get the results in a few days, and that will give us some options of what to do next,' he said kindly. 'I know you'll be out of your mind with worry, Michelle, but dogs can be lumpy, just like people, and some breeds are just more susceptible to them than others. It could very well just be a fatty lump, in which case, it's not likely to cause her any bother at all.'

'So, you would just leave it there?' I asked.

'Absolutely – unless a fatty lump is causing an animal bother, such as affecting their mobility, there's no point taking it out and putting the dog through unnecessary surgery.'

The test had taken less than a minute. Poppy and I went home, but I couldn't stop worrying, no matter what Brian had said. My fingers kept going to the lump. It didn't feel fatty to me, it wasn't squishy, it was what I would call a proper lump – a terrifying one. I'm quite hardy and I'd rather not think of the worst, I tend to feel that you should deal with things in the moment as you never know what will crop up, but I just had a feeling about this. If you are worried or stressed, the dogs pick up on that, so I tried to keep calm.

For the next few days, I was on tenterhooks, desperately trying to reassure myself that it wasn't going to be anything serious. However, when the test results came back, my worst fears were realised.

'We'd like to just check this out,' Brian said. 'Probably best that we give Poppy a biopsy, just to be on the safe side.'

I took her back to the vets, and I couldn't stop the tears pricking my eyes at the thought of there being anything seriously wrong with my beloved Poppy.

Once it was over, I had yet another anxious few days as we waited for the results to come back, but I tried as hard as I could to get on with life as usual. I couldn't just stop my work, but I felt guilty leaving Poppy alone every time I walked out of the door. At night, I held her close to me, but even as she lay there beside me, breathing deeply and contentedly, I couldn't stop my mind from playing out the worst-case scenarios. In the short time she'd been with me, Poppy had become a true lifeline, and I couldn't even begin to imagine what my life would be like without her.

I hoped and prayed that the biopsy results would prove that there was nothing to worry about, but when the vet called me in to discuss the results, all my nightmares came true. The lump was cancerous.

'What do we do now?' I asked Brian.

'We can't leave it – an operation would allow us to remove it and also have a look to see if there was anything else that might be of concern,' he informed me. 'We will also have to cut a bit extra around the lump. If we take away some decent margins then there's much more of a chance that we can get all of the infected area, and that way, the cancer won't spread. It's kind of like scooping it all out.'

There was no other choice to be made really. Poppy had to have the operation. Yes, some cancers can be slow-moving, but I didn't want to risk that. Get it out, check her for any more, then pray she'd be free of it all. The days seemed to crawl by, and by the time the surgery was due, it had turned into September.

Throughout that period, Poppy was her usual precious self, and I kept trying to act normally. 'You'll just have to deal with it on the day,' I told myself. 'Get her to the vets, and trust them. They know what they're doing, they'll do what's best, and all you need to do is keep yourself distracted.'

That was my plan and I stuck to it. Leaving her to have the surgery was horrible, but I was assured that, if everything went according to plan and she recovered well from the anaesthetic, she'd be back with me later that day. I also told myself that, if she'd still been on the street, the lump might not have been picked up on. Even if it had, after the operation, she and Tom would only have had a couple of nights in a Travelodge before being back on the streets. Now that she was with me, I would spoil her rotten once she got home.

My stomach was in knots all day long, and I found that I couldn't focus on anything. My brain just kept drifting back to Poppy, wondering how she was, and whether the surgery would be a success.

As was her way, though, Poppy was an absolute trooper and I collected her late that afternoon, asking Brian, 'How did it all go?'

'Well, we actually found three lumps,' he told me. 'I'm pretty sure two were malignant, and one was nothing to worry about, so we've removed the two cancerous ones and done quite a few tests. She's a sturdy girl, so hopefully that's that. We'll need to have a check-up in a few days, just to make sure the healing process is going well, then she'll get her stitches out next week some time. Just see how she goes and keep her quiet so that she can recover.'

It was a blow to know that there had been more than one lump, but I knew I just had to concentrate on the fact that they thought they'd got it all out and not focus on the risk that that the operation had released cancerous cells into Poppy's body. I had to assume that she was going to get better now, for both of our sakes.

When we got back, Poppy jumped out of the car cautiously and padded into the house where Bailey was waiting for her. I was terrified that she might be in pain, but despite all she'd gone through, she still seemed to have her usual doggy smile on her face, even managing a small tail wag as I let her into the house. As she recovered, Bailey was her protector, barely moving from her side, and he looked after her well. Poppy lay on the sofa while she got over her surgery, and I was beside her all the time. I love the way dogs look at you when you chat to them, and I prattled away all the time to her, hoping that it was helping distract her from the pain in some small way.

Poppy bounced back really well. Street dogs are resil-ient, and without doubt she showed that. Her follow-up check-up went perfectly, and the stitches were removed a few days later. I still talked constantly to Poppy and she still listened. As the days went by though, I couldn't help but notice that she was becoming much greyer around her nose and mouth since the operation – maybe she was feeling the passage of time, as we all do, but now that the cancer had been cut out, I was just hopeful that we still had many years together.

Until she started to cough.

It was maybe about six weeks after her operation, and I wasn't too worried to begin with. I tried a few remedies at home but had to take her back to Brian when they didn't do any good. He thought it was probably just a virus and would pass in time. But it didn't. By November, she was very poorly again – she wasn't her usual self at all. By this point, I was becoming seriously worried. I took her back to Brian again, but he didn't seem concerned at all. He felt sure that it was nothing serious and would pass on its own without medication.

It didn't.

'Come on, Poppy,' I encouraged her every day. 'You need to get this nasty cough out of your system and get yourself better, my lovely.' She'd look at me with those lovely brown eyes which had seen so much, as I willed her to get better, but it just wasn't happening – in fact, it was getting worse.

We returned to the vet yet again, and this time, I was relieved when it was decided to give her a chest x-ray as there was now a suspicion of a chest infection. Antibiotics and steroids were prescribed, and I kept my fingers crossed that we were through the worst of it now, and that Poppy would be back to her old self in no time. But as the days went by, the medicine didn't seem to help at all.

'Oh Pops, you're worrying me so much now – is something else wrong, my love, is it something no one can work out?' It definitely felt that way to me. This didn't seem like a normal cough or a chest infection, and the fact that she was getting worse terrified me. I decided to get a second opinion by going to another vet I also used.

Martin quickly decided that a barrage of blood tests would be required. While we waited for the results, Bailey looked after Poppy, being so sweet and gentle, caring for her as if it was his job – and that made me think there were warning signs that he was picking up on too, maybe something that only another dog would recognise. However, I'm experienced with dogs, I know when it's something that's not serious, and what was going on with Poppy niggled at me day and night. I couldn't shake off a sense of foreboding.

My gut instinct was right. When the results came through, the news was worrying. 'It might indeed be an infection,' he told me, 'but it could also be that the cancer has spread – it might even have gone further before the lumps came out. Let's keep her on steroids for a bit longer as she's terribly wheezy. We'll get her back for an x-ray under anaesthetic if that doesn't work.'

Poppy was struggling, that was clear. Walks were getting shorter every day, and, more worryingly, she wasn't following me around as much or waiting at the door every time I went out. DOTS had a new, much better, mobile van that we'd received in December of that year and, every time I went to try and get things sorted with that, I felt horribly guilty at leaving her. Her eyes were so soulful and they hit me straight in the heart. I wanted to spend every minute with her but I also had so much work to do. Winters were always a particularly hard time for street dogs and their owners and I couldn't expect the volunteers to do everything, no matter how brilliant they were. When I was on DOTS Sunday duty, all I could think of was getting back to Poppy. I knew that Bailey would be taking care of her, but I couldn't bear the thought that she might need me there if she was feeling poorly.

As the days went by, Martin decided that she wasn't actually well enough for an x-ray as the anaesthetic might prove to be problematic with her cough and wheeziness. He upped the steroids and, to my relief, it did help her with her breathing.

'Maybe that's all you needed, Pops,' I told her, rubbing her gorgeous round belly. 'Maybe you just needed something a little stronger to help make that nasty cough go away.'

'Let's check her a week after Christmas and see how she's doing,' Martin suggested. 'It's time for you stop worrying your mum, Poppy – the best Christmas present you could give her would be to get better.'

That calmed me a bit. If we could wait until the week after Christmas, then surely it couldn't be that serious? I just thought that she'd got a nasty infection that she couldn't shake, like those nasty bugs that people get that linger for ages.

Sadly, the steroids weren't as effective as they needed to be and I didn't get the best Christmas gift in the world, which would have been a healthy Poppy. All over that period – Christmas Eve, Christmas Day, Boxing Day – I spent all my time with her, exhorting her to get better.

'Come on, Poppy,' I would whisper into her ear, 'Mummy needs you to be well. You're a tough old thing, just like me – we can do this together.'

She'd smile at me, like always, but she was still getting greyer; there were now flecks of it all over her coat as well as around her nose. I took so many photos and she looked bright in them, posing for the camera, and I just willed us both to get through, get to the week after Christmas when Martin the vet would hopefully work his magic.

FOURTEEN

Gone

Heartbreakingly, the steroids weren't as effective as I had hoped. Instead of waiting for the appointment a week after Christmas, I phoned the vet on the morning of December 28th, unable to wait a moment longer. It had been an awful time; Poppy was listless, clearly not getting any better. Her persona was drained and flat – she wasn't even wagging her tail anymore.

'I need to come in,' I told the receptionist, 'Poppy's not right. Please. Someone has to look at her. I think it's an emergency.'

'OK, bring her in immediately,' they said. 'We'll do her bloods and, if we feel we can do a chest x-ray, we'll go from there.'

I put Poppy in the car, telling her constantly, *We'll get you better, I promise, we'll get you better, Pops.* She always loved looking out of the window from the front seat but she didn't even seem to be interested in that anymore.

When I got her to the surgery, Martin was waiting for us at the door, his face looking very serious.

'Go and get yourself a coffee, Michelle – stay nearby and I'll check her bloods. If she's doing OK, I'll sedate her so that I can get a good look at what's going on.'

'I could just wait here,' I told him, hopefully.

'Find a café, get a coffee. There's no point you hanging around here for ages, fretting about the worst. If she's up to it, I'll sedate her immediately – keep yourself warm and occupied; I'll phone as soon as I can.'

'OK, OK,' I nodded. 'I'll do that.' I bent down towards my Poppy, who managed to wag her tail ever so slightly, as if reassuring me that it was OK for me to go. 'I love you so much, do you know that? Martin is going to make you all better. You'll be back home to cuddles and walks and treats before you know it. Now you be a good girl and Mummy will see you soon. Remember the old saying – we haven't come this far to only come this far.'

Poppy gazed up at me and I swear if she could have talked, she would have told me that she loved me too. I gave her a kiss and a cuddle before leaving the surgery, confirming with the receptionist that they would phone me as soon as they knew what was happening. I didn't care if they thought I was neurotic. This was my Poppy and I needed her back. I found a local café that was open and spent a couple of hours on work calls and checking things for DOTS. All the time, though, my head was with Poppy, wondering what was happening.

Finally, the phone rang and Martin's name flashed up on the screen. I leapt to answer it.

'Hello!' I said on the first ring. 'How is she? Can I get her back? Can I come for Poppy?'

There was a gap before he spoke. A gap that I thought would have been filled with, *It's all OK, Michelle, we did the x-ray and worked it out, she's fine!*

But he didn't say that – and I wasn't prepared for the words I did hear.

'Michelle, you need to come back to the surgery now,' he told me, calmly.

'Why, what's happened? What's going on?' I was panicking.

'I need to talk to you – it's better if you come back to the surgery, Michelle, and we'll chat here.'

'Is she OK? Is Poppy OK?' I pressed.

'Just come back, can you, Michelle? Just come back,' Martin emphasised firmly.

I can't even remember how I got back to the vets, but I did. Martin took me from the reception area to the consultation room – where there was no sign of Poppy. I was sure she'd already died and felt frantic at the thought of losing her.

'Where is she? Where is she?' I wailed.

Martin tried to console me. 'She's resting, Michelle, she's just resting.'

'Oh God, oh God – she's alive then? She's alive?'

'Yes, yes, she is – however . . . Michelle, you need to look at the blood test results.'

He showed me some bits of paper but I had no idea what I was meant to focus on. 'What do they mean?'

Martin took a deep breath and explained. Every blood test was almost zero. Her whole body had crashed.

'I don't know what's keeping her alive,' he told me, shaking his head sadly.

I knew. It was me keeping her alive. It was us. When I think back to that day, in that consulting room, it still gets me. I can smell the spray they clean the surfaces with and hear the phone ringing in reception, all the normal smells and sounds, seeming so ordinary and every day, when in reality, my whole world was crashing down. All I wanted was to get to my Poppy. The numbers from the blood tests were horrific and I didn't know how Martin was going to make her better. All I did know was that I would spend any amount of money, do anything in my power, to keep my dog alive.

'I can't believe it, I can't believe she has more to go through,' I wept. 'After everything she has already coped with, now this – will it be another operation? More than one?'

Martin put his hand on my arm, his eyes kind. 'Michelle – I'm so sorry but we have to let her go.'

'Go? Go? What do you mean "go"?' I honestly think that, by that stage, I had lost the power to process anything. If that had been me with someone else and their dog, I would have dealt with it all efficiently, but this was something else entirely. I didn't want to hear the truth, even though, in my heart, I knew what I had to do.

'Poppy's body is riddled with cancer. If you take her home, she will die a terrible, struggling death. You adore her, Michelle. You don't want that for her.' I was gasping for breath as he spoke, tears rolling down my cheeks. 'I'll get the nurse to bring Poppy through and you spend as much time as you need with her. Then we'll make sure she's at peace.'

When she came through that door, her tail wagging just as much as it used to, I fell to the floor. Holding her in my arms, all I could say, over and over again was, *I'm so sorry, I'm so sorry.*

She was only eight years old. I had thought I would have her for twice that time; we'd been together for such a little while and I had so much love to give her. This was cruel but keeping her for my own benefit would be even worse. I told her that I had to let her go, the words choking me as they came out. I think she knew. I think Poppy knew this was it. We were together for an hour and it was as if she was comforting me. I lay there whispering to her, telling her how much she meant to me, and what a difference she had made to my life. I promised her I would never forget her, and I promised her I would keep her legacy going forever. She smiled, she wagged her tail, she snuggled into me. We squeezed as much love as we could into that hour.

Martin kept coming in to check on me, and on more than one occasion he shook his head in disbelief, staring down at her. 'I just can't believe how this dog has kept on going.'

It took me back to when I had first seen her in the police kennel. How, from that first meeting when we had found each other, it had given us both so much. Now we were at the end together and there hadn't been much time at all. I knew that Poppy had taught me so much and given me such a lot; I knew that I had taken her off the streets and done a lot for her too, but it would never be enough. She was the most wonderful dog and I didn't know how I would ever go home again to a house that didn't have her waiting for me at the door.

At last, Martin came back in and said, 'It's time, Michelle.'

I knew that I couldn't hold her forever and that this was the last act of love I could perform for my Poppy. All of us who have been in that situation know how horrendous it is, your heart breaking in two as you say goodbye for the last time, but for their sake, you have to smile at them, you have to let them know that this is fine, everything is just as it should be.

I felt the vet gently take my hand from Poppy's head as I said, *I love you* over and over again. There wasn't enough time to tell her how much I adored her – there never would be. As Martin got the syringe ready and I looked at Poppy's beautiful, trusting face, I experienced a flash of clarity.

I couldn't be here.

I couldn't stay with her for this.

I wanted to remember her as the spirited girl she was, not dying. I didn't want to remember Poppy as the life faded from her body, I wanted to remember her full of bounce and happiness. If I'd stayed, the memory I would have for as long as I lived would be of my wonderful girl, lifeless.

'I can't do it,' I whispered to Martin. 'I can't be here when she goes.'

I kissed her one last time and walked out of that room. I knew she was in good hands with Martin and the nurse. I didn't want to say goodbye to her, I didn't want that to be my last memory of her. Just as I was leaving the room, I looked back. Poppy looked at me and I just knew in that moment that it wasn't a goodbye. I ran outside with her lead and collar in my hands, and in all honesty felt a crushing guilt. Had I been weak? Had I let her down? I didn't know, I truly didn't know in those first moments. I was in shock. I'd gone to the vets that morning thinking it could all be sorted and now, unbelievably, I was leaving without her.

I barely remember getting home, but as soon as I got inside, I felt as though I just wanted to stay there forever. I went to bed and cried, snuggling against the blankets that still had a faint scent of Poppy. The only thing I had the strength for was to call and request a private cremation. I carried the weight of my guilt for the first two days, feeling listless and subdued. I couldn't stand the thought of never seeing my darling girl again.

But one day, I woke up feeling a little lighter. I was lying awake, watching the sunrise, as I realised an incredible thing – I *would* see her again. When we both met at Rainbow Bridge, whenever that was, Poppy would be waiting for me and we would be by each other's side for all eternity. I think it was that which made me realise I couldn't wallow. What would be the point of Poppy's loss if I just gave up? There were dogs out there who needed help, I had an organisation that she would want me to keep going – I doubted I would have had the strength to keep going if I'd seen her put to sleep as I would only have had that image in my mind.

I felt that Poppy was telling me to get up and get going. It spurred me on to think that she wanted me to do this. When our dogs pass, they may not be with you in fur, but they'll always be with you in spirit and soul. I believe that last moment at the vet's wasn't goodbye. I'm a very spiritual person and I slowly made sense of the fact – and it was fact to me – that Poppy had only passed from this earthly plane. Her spirit was still with me, and she'd be beside me wherever I walked.

For the first few days after Poppy was put to sleep, my other dogs didn't seem to notice, but there was a point when Bailey definitely began to look for Poppy. I buried my face into his soft fur, knowing he missed her just as I did. Ten days after she passed, I received her ashes back in a beautiful gunmetal urn with her pawprint and name on it. I placed her collar around it and put it by my bed. *Now you'll be with me while I sleep too, Poppy. We'll rest together.* A friend brought me a Rainbow Bridge candle holder and, to this day, when I get home, I always light a candle for Poppy.

Was I bitter about her passing so young? No, I don't think so, but I did desperately wish that she had been allowed to stay a little longer. I've seen Staffies twice her age on the streets, but I did hate to think about what her death would have been like if she had still been living rough with Tom. As it was, she had everything, I was the one who was bereft. She was a spiritual dog who was with me for a reason. I believe that animals come here for a purpose. They go to the people who need them. For a while, that person for Poppy had been Tom; then she knew that I needed her more. When you want a dog, don't look; they'll find you just as Poppy found me. I felt that she saw me for who I was; she was my counsellor and she'd lick my tears away, and I had to acknowledge the loss of that, even while still believing we'd meet again.

I'd say to anyone who has lost a pet, or who is facing the loss of one, you must grieve their loss. It's part of healing – but don't just grieve that they've gone, think of what you still have with them. Your routine will change, there will be no walks together, no cuddles on the sofa, but they're there, just in a different way. I still put three bowls down for Bailey, Milly and Poppy. I sometimes lay out an extra dentastick to let her know she is still in my mind and that I want to treat her. She was an incredibly powerful dog who completely redirected my life. Before, I did plenty of things and I was content, but I'd never felt the true passion that she inspired in me. Poppy changed everything, and I would have been diminishing this if I fell apart completely.

In my mind, grieving the loss of an animal is the same as grieving for a human. You still have to go through the same stages. First, there is shock and denial – *how can this have happened? How can I be without her?* Next, there is often anger; you feel bitter and resentful. *Why did this happen to me, to my dog? Why did I have so little time with her when there was still so much love to share?* If you have faith, you can lose it at this point, because if there was really a god, someone or something out there, why would they put you through this? There is frustration and anger and guilt for such a long time. The third stage is bargaining – *did I make the right deci-sion?* Even when there was no decision to be made, even when it was taken out of your hands. You bargain in your mind, you would do anything to have them back again, anything. This has nothing to do with reality – you know it won't happen, but the need to find a solution to getting your beloved animal back with you is still in your head. This can move to a fourth stage, low mood or even depression, as you realise that it won't work, that there is nothing to bargain with; it's just fact that they are gone and the deep, dragging reality of feeling like it will last forever. Finally, acceptance, realising that it *has* happened, that maybe you can move on and that there were wonderful things about the time you did have together. It isn't easy to get to this place, and I don't believe you ever forget or fully recover, but you do learn to live with it.

I know that there may be people reading this who are in the throes of grief, who may have lost their beloved pet recently, and I want you to try and take comfort from the love you shared. No one knew the full truth of how perfect your relationship was, and you will feel that there isn't a single person in the world who could understand, so what I would suggest is that you give yourself time to think of those wonderful moments and cry as much as you want. Don't keep it in – why should you? Weep and wail and scream if you want to. They have gone and you should be allowed to express it any way you want.

For others, reading this might bring back so much. You might have lost a pet when you were a child, you might have had a dog who lived until it was twenty and that might have been some time ago . . . it's OK to still grieve. I'll know that I'll never forget Poppy if I live to be a hundred.

The sorrow comes in waves, often when we least expect it, and that's normal. Animals take up a special place in our hearts and that place will frequently remind us of its presence, often at the strangest times.

Wherever you are in your grief, however you respond, however long it has been, it's fine to feel what you feel.

Other people may not understand because to them it's just an animal – but for you, they *were* family, not just part of the family. Talk about them, never block them out. Your animal was there to bring peace, love and joy and connection, and you shouldn't deny that. It doesn't matter how they go – death is death. It's the fact that they aren't part of your life any longer that gives you this sense of tremendous loss. If you knew you could just get them back for a little while, maybe that would be OK, maybe you would cope better, but ultimately, you would always have to say goodbye at some point. I'm not an expert, I can't tell people the definitive way to grieve – all I can say is that you should give yourself time and space and try not to feel guilty. Connect with people who have the same outlook and feelings about animals. Do things in their memory. (I went to the park and took a big box of tennis balls as a gift to other dogs from Poppy!)

I really do believe that the promise of Rainbow Bridge can keep us going. Your animal lets you know when it's time and Poppy's light had gone out. We feel guilty making the decision, but they've already made it. She made me go to the vet that day as she was so different, so flat and not herself, as if she was saying, *If you don't take me today, it will be awful for both of us*. The spiritual part of me knows that there is a time to live and a time to die. I believe that animals have an innate wisdom that allows them to know this better than we do. All we can focus on is loving them and helping them on their way when it all gets too much. It's the last thing we can do for them and although it hurts like hell, there does come a day when you smile more than you cry.

Even though Poppy has gone, she left me with a reason to continue my street dog work. After all, she had been mine, but she had been a street dog too, originally. I could be negative, I could weep forever (and believe me, I often felt that that was the option I wanted), but DOTS was to be her legacy. I was determined to expand it and make sure I could get as many street dogs supported as possible.

FIFTEEN

Poppy's legacy

DOTS had to grow – this would be Poppy's legacy. On the streets, dogs' needs would rarely be met, as Poppy's had been in her time of need. I would have to be their voice. I'd have to shout louder than I'd ever shouted before. That was fine – I had the lungs and the determination for it! Ideally, eventually, I wanted to expand to different areas of the UK, to reach more people and more dogs.

I was a woman on a mission. Poppy would not be forgotten and her name would live on. This was her charity; I'd simply run it for her. A few people had known I had Tom's dog, but I really only told my team of volunteers about Poppy's passing. I'd never taken her with me to the station on The Strand; in fact, she'd never been back to Central London since I'd got her as I worried that it might be traumatic for her. My team was amazing, really supportive, and they knew how deeply I was affected, but I had no plans to speak about my loss with clients. I had to focus.

Poppy died on the Thursday and I was back with the van on the Sunday, New Year's Eve. I felt different. Normally when I met up with my team, they would ask how I was, but now they knew not to fuss, even though I wasn't my normal chirpy self. They took over all the conversations and got me through the day. We saw twelve dogs that day, which was about right – any amount between ten and twenty were arriving on Sundays by this stage.

I kept taking a look at one of the last photos of Poppy on my phone – her eyes looked brighter than they had for weeks, and that was a sign for me. It was going to be my inspiration.

Is that it, Poppy? I wondered, looking at the photo. *Have I got to get a move on?*

I could see her smiling at me in my mind's eye, never taking her gaze off me for a second, just as she always had.

Right then, I told her. *Let's really get this going. Let's see just how far we can take this thing.*

Poppy was right. It was time.

I had my street work to do, and I needed to open more stations – I knew this as clearly as if Poppy was shouting it to me. On 6 January 2018, we opened our street station in Oxford, followed by Chatham, Milton Keynes, Taunton and Bournemouth. I worked as hard as I could to open as many as possible. Most stations were available once a month, but I was permanently exhausted.

I also decided that DOTS would also help people in areas we didn't cover; we'd find a vet practice and cover the cost. I was running on love for Poppy, answering my phone constantly, messaging, chasing things up, never settling, on the go almost 24/7. What everyone wants for their dog is the same: vet care, nutritious food, foster care if needed, and love. I did everything in my power to tick all the items on that list.

One night, I was doing outreach work in Victoria. My heart was still broken from the loss of Poppy – I couldn't imagine a day when it wouldn't be – but I had the conviction that she had brought me to this point, and there was no way I would ever let her down. There would always be dogs on the streets that I needed to help, and my Poppy would be looking over me every minute I spent doing that.

Come on, darling, I said to her in my mind, as usual. *Plenty for us to be doing, no point in wallowing.*

To be honest, it wasn't any different to all the other nights I'd worked. I was chatting to the people I knew, making sure they had what they needed and that the dogs were all OK. To be honest, it was one of those sessions where everybody was pretty much all right, there more for the opportunity to just talk rather than actually asking for help that would keep them going. Everyone seemed quite settled, the weather was all right, so I decided to move on to my next stage, looking out for any new street homeless and their dogs.

As I was wandering about, I could see three men coming down the road towards me. Two of them were walking in a completely nondescript way, but there was something about the third guy, a very tall man, which made me hesitate. Something about the way he walked was familiar. They got closer and all of a sudden, it hit me.

I'm sure that's Poppy's dad! I thought. *That's Tom!*

The other guys were chatting away, but Tom was just walking between them, staring at the ground, which meant he couldn't see me coming towards him.

He was only a few steps away from me when he finally raised his head.

'Ah, Michelle!' was all he said, before putting his arms around me and wrapping me in a loving hug. I was so glad to see him, the man who had brought the most amazing dog into my world.

He moved back a little, still with his hands on my arms, and smiled.

'How's my Poppy?' he asked.

I felt as if there was ice in my veins. Oh my God. They hadn't told him.

'Tom,' I said, softly, 'you didn't hear?'

'Hear what?'

'I am so sorry – did they not tell you?'

I could see the colour drain from his face as he whispered his reply.

'Tell me what?'

'Oh Tom – Poppy passed away.'

For a moment I thought he was going to collapse, but we both had to be strong.

'After she died, Tom, I reached out to your caseworker and told her. I begged her to get in touch and let you know. She said that you had moved on and that she couldn't discuss anything about you with me, couldn't tell me where you were, couldn't give me any contact details for you. But she promised, Tom, she promised. I told her that I wanted to let you know about how much she was loved, and I gave the caseworker my number just in case you didn't have it. I never heard anything back but I was sure she would have told you about your girl. Our girl.'

Tom was nodding throughout all of this, but the tears were pouring down his face uncontrollably, and he looked heartbroken.

I just held him.

It was all I could do.

When he finally stopped weeping, he said something which meant the world to me.

'I'm so happy that she spent that time with you, Michelle. I feel that you would have done anything for her.'

'Tom, I need you to absolutely know that Poppy meant the world to me. I loved her with every bone in my body and if anything could have been done to keep her with me, I would have moved mountains. Honestly, I believe that when I met you, and I met Poppy, that it was all for a reason.'

He nodded, still holding onto me, and though he still looked distraught, he had stopped crying now.

'Do you know what she's done?' I asked him. 'Do you know what her legacy is?'

I began to tell him all about DOTS, that we had a street station with a vet van which ran nose-to-tail checks for dogs. I told him about our registered vet and the fact that, as a result of having that vet, we were now a registered vet practice ourselves. I told him about our full triage team, our access to dog trainers, groomers and nutritionists, that we gave food, advice, collars, leads, waterproofs, a one-stop shop for every street dog who came our way. He looked stunned by it all. I told him about how his little girl (or not so little!) had inspired me to set up the organisation and about how she would never be forgotten. I could see that it meant so much to him, and, actually, as I recounted the whole story to him, I could feel a shift in me too . . .

Poppy was by my side, I knew that – but, I also knew that she had taken me to her dad that night. In all that time, I had never seen Tom and now she had made sure we crossed paths. It was an emotional moment when Tom and I went our separate ways that night, and my head was spinning. There was something in this, there was a lesson Poppy was trying to teach me.

I knew that she was there.

I knew that she had decided it was time for her dad and her mum to meet again.

I knew that Tom needed to know that she had passed.

I *knew* all of that – so, what was I missing?

I have said many times that I believe dogs come to us for a reason. They know the point in our life when we will need them, and they know that there is something they need to teach us. Telling Tom had been awful, but I actually realised why it had happened, why Poppy had decided it had to be that night.

It was time.

It was time for me to say goodbye to the final part of Poppy. A shiver ran through me as I realised it was almost as if the circle had closed. I'd told Tom about the legacy she'd left, and I needed to understand that for myself too. I couldn't grieve forever. When you lose a pet, it can be the most devastating thing in the world. The way you feel about them never leaves you, but there has to come an acceptance of the fact that they have left this level of our experience. I believe they are still there, but I also believe that they would want us to realise that we can't stand still forever.

What I feel more than anything is that there is an honesty, a rawness to existence on the streets, which had already given me purpose. With Poppy's help, with her still beside me, I had found my purpose. I knew how it felt to be invisible, because that had been my own way of life for years. I wanted to give homeless people a voice because I'd never had one. I did all I could for the day-to-day existence of street dogs but I also wanted to be part of something which created pathways to the rehabilitation of their owners. With such a high incidence of mental health or addiction problems – or often both – I really wanted to help people tackle their demons with their dogs by their side. Why should they have to choose? As I'd seen so many times, many had turned down housing or any accommodation when offered because it wasn't dog-friendly. For others, separation wasn't something that could be predicted – just like Tom and Poppy. Illness or hospitalisation generally came without warning, which meant that I would have to be able to provide free foster care at a moment's notice. I needed to think of all angles and I needed to aim high.

As I've mentioned, street dog owners tended to be single men and they were the hardest to accommodate through council channels. This group is the most prone to homelessness, due to marriage breakdown, unemployment or landlords kicking them out. Often the housing crisis is to blame – there is limited social housing, and a lot of private landlords don't welcome dogs. These animals are invaluable, I had found out, when their owners had fast unravelling mental health issues, so why would anyone in their right minds think that separation was a good idea? People are so quick to make assumptions. The bond between these owners and their dogs is inextricable. One is nothing without the other. The dog is their lifeline and I had to continuously commit to doing everything in my power to ensure that that bond, that lifeline, was maintained and strengthened.

When I got home that night, I went straight back to making lists – in summer we needed more supplies of oral rehydration drinks, water, cooling coats, caps for humans, and a place for dogs to rest if they were really struggling. We'd take temperatures and monitor heart rates if we had to. Public concern can be high during cold spells, but heat-waves are just as dangerous. When dogs have heatstroke, it can be fatal. In winter, we still needed piles of socks, piles of blankets, and piles of warm coats for both dogs and owners. Most homeless people are clued up about their animals and in difficult weather tend to put their dog's needs first. I had started to give out rucksacks with everything they would need for both parties when they were on the move, including orange and black bandanas to show they were a DOTS dog!

A lot of homeless people have a tendency not to mix well with others – which might be because of abuse or mental health problems – and I would always tell them, *You sort your life out and I'll sort the dog out.* I realised I would do anything for those animals, just as I would do anything for my own. I paid for doggy funerals, I paid for hotels when they needed them. As police cells don't accept dogs, I would sometimes have to rush to a police station in the middle of the night to collect Fido or whoever needed a last-minute place to stay. I was still on call, day and night, seven days a week, and I knew that I always would be. Most services for the homeless close at 5 p.m. but homeless lives don't run to a timetable.

Putting all of my heart and soul into running DOTS consumed me after Poppy's death and for the next year or so. I had to think of everything. Over that time, I like to think that I was able to provide people with stability and consistency. They could turn up freely with a hundred and one questions, and they knew I would always be there with my team if they needed something. Perhaps just as importantly, the DOTS stations had also become somewhere people could come and socialise as well, and interact with those they didn't necessarily want to chat to on the street.

The real moments of joy for me, and when I knew DOTS had made a real impact, were when we saw the same dog coming back week after week. One such dog was Gunner, a real Heinz 57 who I first got to know on the street and then through the mobile vet van. His owner, Justin, really struggled with getting food consistency for Gunner and was also paranoid that someone was going to take his dog away. We would try to reassure him, telling him exactly what he needed to do to take care of his dog, in a way that meant no one would have any grounds to complain. Unfortunately, though, a lot of street people take any suggestion to be a criticism, so you have to do it in a certain way.

Justin was always very protective of Gunner, and was constantly terrified that he wasn't doing well, or that something was wrong, or that someone was going to take the dog away from him. It's vitally important for us to build up a trusting relationship with both human and animal, giving advice without making someone feel patronised or humiliated and ultimately pushing them away. As the days and weeks went by, we managed to help Justin to access good food for Gunner and, as the trust developed, medical support too. It didn't happen overnight, though. Often, all it takes is for people to realise that someone believes in them. The truth was that Justin was actually a fantastic owner, but he had to be shown how good he was. A few months later, the pair managed to find accommodation together, and it was a joy to see how far they had come in such a short space of time.

It was very humbling, and also exciting, that the word was spreading. The dogs now coming to us weren't just from the Westminster area anymore; people were starting to come to us from all across the city. I'd thrown myself in at the deep end and such was the demand for DOTS services, I was still learning on my feet about addiction, mental health, abuse and the myriad other issues that people face when living on the streets. It was quite surreal really, and I didn't always know what I was doing. This had all grown from an idea I'd had all those years ago when I saw Kenneth outside Waitrose and decided I would help street people with dogs. From simply providing the basics, Poppy had taught me that I needed to do more, go further to help meet these dogs' needs. The vet, the groomer, the trainer, people to help, all of that had just developed as and when it was needed. I didn't have any idea where it was going to go; I had no real plan, just a desire to make a difference. I never in a million years dreamed that, in three short years, we would have come this far, launching and successfully running DOTS, and I hadn't really absorbed it.

It had truly been a whirlwind, and I felt as though I'd barely stopped in the year or so since Poppy had passed. Finally, I took a breath. I had to take a look back at all that we'd done. There had been a lot of highs, but also a hell of a lot of lows. Whilst it was incredibly rewarding work, and whilst the media coverage, awards and accolades we received were welcomed, it was also exhausting, because the exposure brought with it new people who badly needed our support, and we were also stretched to our very limits. It was at that time that we also needed to raise awareness in order to get funding because our expenditure was increasing at such a fast rate. Everyone on the project was a volunteer and I needed to look at how we could sustain this. The issues were always going to be there. It wasn't as if, suddenly, one day there would be no dogs on the streets; this meant I had to get a long-term plan in place. I had to think big.

Come on Michelle, I told myself. *It's time to think big again. You've done it before, and Poppy is there to guide you. What do they need now, what can DOTS do that will change everything?*

It would come. I knew it. The idea would come.

SIXTEEN

Roxy

While I was waiting on my big idea from Poppy, normal life – as normal as it ever was – continued.

Roxy was a Staffie cross who had been one of our very first clients. She was there on the opening day of DOTS, back in March 2017, and it was always a joy to see her. Roxy belonged to a rough sleeper called Liam, whose stomping ground was Tottenham Court Road. I'd known him prior to starting DOTS, when I first started doing outreach work. Back then, I had told Liam my idea of setting up this new service, but at that time it was one that I couldn't guarantee would work. However, Liam was very supportive.

'God, Michelle, I feel quite overwhelmed by this,' he had said. 'You do so much for the dogs already. People see that there is some stuff for us, soup kitchens, caseworkers, that sort of thing, but they never think of the dogs. There's nothing for them. You're one of a kind, you are.'

'Ah, you'll make me blush,' I laughed. 'It's really the dogs who have taught me everything I know. Watching them, being with them, they make it clear what they need and I just have to find a way to get it all in place.' It was true. I would never have worked all of this out without the help of the dogs, particularly Poppy.

Roxy was a sprightly dog for her age, probably about eight years old, just like my Poppy had been – it's hard to know what age street dogs are because their owners don't have much concept of time either. I have no idea how Liam had got her as I never ask questions like that. People come to the services I provide for a reason and they don't like being questioned. Probing them about where the dog came from or what their background is doesn't matter, it's irrelevant, they need help in the here and now; there's no benefit to anyone raking over their past. They're there and they need help, I would always tell them, 'Let's move forward, not back.'

Liam did give me a few snippets of his past life though – I knew that he'd had Roxy during one of his 'indoor' periods; she wasn't a dog that he'd just acquired when he began rough sleeping. Liam had been on and off the streets for a while, with Roxy at his side all her life. In fact, he'd been homeless on and off for thirty or forty years, so I assumed there had been a few dogs over that period. Liam had an alcohol addiction, which got worse the longer he was on the streets, so every time he went inside to accommodation, he would find it harder and harder to settle. The only way he could really get help for himself was if it was street-based, because of his unwillingness and inability to leave Roxy.

Up until I found him, probably 99.9 per cent of daytime services wouldn't let dogs in. That was changing slightly now, since DOTS had broken the mould, and more services were starting to see how important it was that the dogs were there; that it's vital not only for the client but for the dog too – they just can't be separated. I knew that there was still a lot of work to do with daytime services in that regard, and I would need to keep plugging away.

Liam had, at one point, also had a partner who was rough sleeping. It was a volatile relationship, which added to his revolving doors attitude between street life and accommodation. He was a stubborn character and put up huge barriers to accepting help. It wasn't that he was bad or wrong– he just didn't want to engage with the services, and used to say that the street was his home. There could have been support for Liam but, unfortunately, he became very institutionalised, which can happen to rough sleepers, as they become deeply psychologically attached to the pavements they bed down on, and the city they walk through every day. On top of that, his addiction made things very difficult and I would find him completely knocked out and oblivious some days, Roxy by his side, watchful and protective.

'Is your dad not with it again?' I'd ask her. 'I'll come back later then, girl. You stand guard and have a few treats on me.' I'd leave her, happily munching on some chewy nibbles, knowing that Liam couldn't have a better angel looking out for him.

As daunting as the street is, it's a very sociable environment for these people when they're together and if they want to be part of a little group. Liam used to sleep outside Heals department store, with his rucksack, which we had provided, and his sleeping bag. Roxy was his reason for living, his absolute everything. They were very well known in the Westminster area with their amazing partnership. They lived for each other and she was a very happy girl. Every time I saw her, she'd be wagging her tail and smiling in that typical Staffie way, and I knew that – despite what a lot of people passing by might think – she was living her best life as long as she was with Liam. He really lived for her; he stayed on the streets for her, as he could have accessed permanent accommodation if he gave her up. She was always looking at him, with both of them very wary of everyone outside of their little bubble. Liam looked after Roxy, and Roxy looked after him, that was clearly evident. She was a reason to get up in the morning and to find a safe space to bed down at night. A lot of street people who live without dogs don't really have a reason.

Roxy and Liam always had the bare essentials like food; it was just that Liam could only rely on what he got at any one time. Coming to DOTS gave him the consistency that had been missing, and that was what he was grateful for. Not only that, it gave him somewhere to be. He and Roxy enjoyed the socialising aspect of things with us. It wasn't just about coming and getting what they needed; it was very much all of the interaction, and to regularly see people they trusted.

'I can't tell you how much I enjoy being here,' Liam told me one Sunday. 'You don't know what a relief it is to know that I can come here and be myself. You treat me like a normal person, not just another person on the street, in the gutter, who has nothing.'

I heard that a lot; it was the feedback we received across the board from those who used our services, and it was especially true with Liam as I had such a good rapport with him. He trusted me, and he just enjoyed coming along. Once he'd come once or twice, we came to know that, come rain or shine, he'd be there waiting for us, would always offer to help unload the van, set everything up and spend the most time with us every week, while others came and went as and when. Not only was he the first one there, he was the last one to leave. I knew it was partly because of his Roxy, because she loved all the fuss she got, not to mention the treats, but partially because it was his way of giving back. By helping us, he felt valued and valuable.

Liam might have been struggling with alcohol addiction, but he was also a great guy. He was funny; a typical Scot who could talk to anyone. He also loved to draw and was always drawing in chalk on the pavement where the van was. His artwork always caused people to and look and compliment his work, which gave him a purpose as well. When he drew, it was never pictures of his beloved Roxy though; it would be things that encouraged passers-by to support DOTS. He was looking to give back to us because we were giving so much to him and Roxy. I felt touched by how much he contributed in the ways that he could.

On days he felt really down, we were there to pick him up. I used to make a point of going to see him during the week, taking him coffee and cake, which he loved, and treats for Roxy. We'd just sit and talk on the street. It could be about anything – the cars passing by, the people we saw and their imaginary lives, or it could be about films, books or just generally about how we were both feeling, because he used to care about how I was, too. I tried not to focus on his situation because I already knew about it and knew what we could and couldn't change, but he was kind, and interested and interesting. Liam was a great guy, but it was sad to know that he was also very troubled.

Dogs on the street don't have a favourite anything, so Roxy didn't have a favourite treat, but she was happy with anything, that was just her nature. Dogs living on the streets have such an inconsistent diet and sadly, they can't always have something they want. We can't guarantee to give them the same treats every week – we always try to give them the same food as much as we can, but treats vary.

I also ask people not to give the dogs too many treats as they're very fattening.

Roxy loved people, loved the company, and was amazingly loyal to Liam. She always got very excited when she saw me and would run up the street to me, because, like all the dogs, they get to know you. She was a really sweet, gentle, lovely girl who had adapted to street life incredibly well, but she was feeding off that comfort from Liam because he was very experienced and relaxed on the street. Street dogs are rarely bundles of anxiety and Roxy really just went with the flow. If Liam had to go around the corner to wee, she would sit in one place, she wouldn't move – she was never a wanderer, all she wanted to do was wait for her dad to come back. Street dogs are people-orientated; basically, lots of people approach them out on the street and they have to be calm. As time went on, Roxy just got to know the team – us – more and more, but she'd always been completely adaptable, like most street dogs. They also love the attention. They're little flirts, really!

Everyone got used to seeing Roxy and Liam every week, and they felt like a key part of our routine. It was a rare occasion that Liam was late or didn't show up, and if he didn't arrive, we would wonder if he was OK. If I hadn't seen him that day, the next day I would make a point of going to where I knew he was likely to be, watching the world go by. Often it was that he had had a drink and didn't know what day it was, never mind the time. If any of my regulars didn't show up one week, I'd make a call if they had a phone, or either go and check if they were OK or ask someone else to do it.

One Sunday, when we got to The Strand, Liam was waiting as usual. He rushed straight over as soon as we'd parked and said, 'Look Michelle, something's not right with Roxy!'

'What is it?' I asked. 'Is she sick?'

'Yes, she can't eat, can't seem to hold her food down, and she's staggering about.'

I looked down at Roxy and my heart broke for the beautiful girl. It was clear that Liam was right to be concerned. There was something very wrong with her indeed. Our vet hadn't arrived yet, so I rushed Roxy and Liam to the nearest vet I knew of who did charity work. The vet examined Roxy and shook his head. It was clear that she was very poorly indeed, and the vet announced that she would need to see a specialist. I knew that DOTS would be fine with the volunteers that day – Roxy was my priority. Thankfully, the vet had called ahead, and she was admitted straight away. The specialist carried out some tests and the diagnosis came through quickly.

Roxy had a brain tumour, affecting the front part of her brain. It had been developing for a long time, and it was too late to operate. Basically, there was no hope for that beautiful girl, and she would have to be put to sleep. It was like Poppy all over again. Liam was devastated, and I felt the pain of Poppy's loss coursing through me as I saw the tragedy repeating itself.

'Is she going? Is she leaving me?' he asked, his eyes wide with fear.

The vet was very kind and patient, and told Liam that he could take her for one more day together but then the only option would be for him to let her go. The flashbacks to Poppy were distressing, but I was very upset about Roxy too, as I loved that dog. The thought of her not running along Tottenham Court Road when she caught sight of me was almost too much to bear, but I had to be strong for her and for Liam.

'I just want a normal day with her,' Liam whispered to me as we left. 'Nothing special.'

'It will be special though,' I told him. 'You'll be with her and she'll be with you. What could be more special than that?'

I know that they just went back to their usual haunts. He took Roxy to say 'goodbye' to a few street friends, and even sat on their usual spot on Tottenham Court Road. Roxy wasn't really up to doing much more anyway, but those last hours together, padding about, going to a little park and loving each other meant the world to Liam.

The next day, the vet had made a really lovely area for Roxy to be put to sleep in, with cosy blankets and a candle burning for her. Our DOTS groomer was there too, and the three of us said our goodbyes and spoke softly to her as she passed. I arranged for her pawprints to be taken and for her to be cremated.

'We'll have a service for her at the station,' I told Liam as I held his weeping body, wracked with the pain of losing his beloved girl. 'We'll never forget our Roxy.'

I wasn't altogether surprised when Liam disappeared for a little while after Roxy had gone. I suspected that he just couldn't cope with visiting the station without Roxy, a place he associated so much with his precious dog. His alcohol addiction spiralled out of control and, every time I went to find him, he would be crying, sobbing non-stop as he recounted stories about his life with Roxy. It was really hard to witness. It was clear that Liam simply felt he had no reason to carry on anymore. Roxy was his sole purpose in life, and without her, he felt he had no reason to get up anymore, he had no reason to live. Losing his dog was the worst thing in the world that could have happened to him. I tried to encourage him to come back to the station to help us out; I told him how much he was missed and that we would have another little ceremony there to commemorate Roxy if he could just bring himself to come along.

'I'll try Michelle, I'll try, but my world is empty without her. I can't imagine why I even bother being here.'

The next Sunday, I set up a small table with a picture of Roxy and some candles illuminating the image of her beautiful face. As I was putting the finishing touches to it, I felt a hand on my shoulder.

It was Liam.

'I can't thank you enough, Michelle,' he cried. 'She'll be remembered, won't she? No one will forget my girl.'

'Of course, we won't, Liam. Not now, and not ever. She was a brilliant, precious dog, and we will never, ever forget her.'

He found it all really emotional, but thankfully, I think it did help. As people stopped by, they would ask about the picture, and the beautiful dog. Liam was proud of her and told them that she was his baby, that was his Roxy. Passers-by were lovely to him and all gave Liam their condolences. He couldn't stop talking about DOTS and how much we'd supported him and his girl, giving a little speech about what a beautiful dog she was and the huge part she had played in his life. He also spoke about how much he, as well as Roxy, used to enjoy coming to us.

It was at the station that we sprinkled her ashes. Liam clung onto the urn as if he was holding Roxy, and we all cried that day. I told him that I would have a bracelet made with some of the ashes in for him so he would always have her close.

It devastated me. It's horrendous to lose such a beautiful dog who had meant so much to me and my team, but it's also utterly heartwrenching to see the owner so broken by the loss. I felt helpless for a while, not knowing what we could do to help Liam. It was very sad indeed until we managed to pull it all back a little with the ceremony.

By this stage, DOTS was definitely becoming more recognised. We'd received a lot of interest from the press and the media, and if it helped spread the word about the work we were doing and raised awareness of the reality of life on the streets, that could only be a good thing. Media coverage helped to highlight a service that was much needed. We were very surprised at how open people were to what we were doing, and I always tried to organise things which would get a bit of attention. In the summer months at the station we used to have a swimming pool, and, once a month, we would do a themed event such as a paw party. This was a tea party for the dogs where I would make them bowls of doggy tea and plates of doggy cakes – everyone loved that and lots of tourists would stop and take photos! I'd have Easter parties, Christmas parties, anything that would get the DOTS name out there and let people know about the important services we provided.

We grew quite quickly, and thankfully other groups started to try to get services to accept dogs too. I always looked forward to Sundays, to seeing everybody, meeting new dogs and engaging with people. It was a pleasure to see the same faces coming along every week, and it made me feel that people felt safe with us; they liked coming to us, and most importantly of all, they trusted us with their most prized possession, their dog. As street people can be very guarded and don't let others in very easily, it was even more rewarding to have these regular attendees, even if they just popped in to say 'hello'.

We were flying, and it was all because of Poppy.

SEVENTEEN

The Sanctuary

I still used to talk to Poppy every time I came home, telling her about my good day or my bad day. 'What have you done?' I'd say to her.

I had a stunning wire creation made of her in January 2019 as I wanted to remember her more visibly as well as in my heart, to make sure she was always waiting for me when I came home.

I loved and missed my baby girl so much. On the anniversary of her death, I wrote on our DOTS page:

Poppy taught me everything about street dogs, especially the Staffie breed, and she was the most loving, loyal and appreciative dog I knew. She'd nose-nudge my other pawjuss fur family away if they invaded her snuggle time with me, she'd follow me everywhere and I felt so loved and protected. My world fell apart the morning she so devastatingly passed away after becoming very poorly from cancer. I remember taking her to the vet for a check-up and coming home with just her lead and collar and tears running down my face. I promised her I will forever look after her FUR-iends on the street and her legacy lives on. RIP, my beautiful baby that is forever in my mind and heart.

I wanted everyone to know just what she had done for me. I felt that I always had a bit of street life at home with Poppy. She made me understand that way of living more, even though I'd already been doing my outreach work for five years, but I think you can only truly comprehend the life of the homeless when you see the harsh realities. It hits hard. When Tom said she should be with me, I always felt like I had a little bit of the street under my own roof.

I was never detached from my work on the streets; it wasn't a job from which you could come home and switch off. I just felt as if street life, with these people and their dogs, was my life. Poppy gave me an insight into all of it – the life, the dogs, especially the Staffie breed, their personalities. She gave me that window through which I could see how rough sleepers felt about their dogs, and that bond. I knew that the incredible love I had for Poppy must have been tenfold for an owner who had nothing else in the world. Street dogs are just such different dogs. Their whole being; everything about them is so different from a normal pet. Their love and loyalty can hardly be described. I couldn't walk around the house without her next to me. I never had to call her and she gave me such a sense of feeling really wanted, of being loved and protected. It's such an amazing thing to experience and

I felt so very lucky that I'd managed to have that with Poppy.

The street people have always been very kind to me, so supportive. It's not about me, even if they say I'm their angel, it's about them and their companions. They are intensely private people – like me – but I do like to think they see me as a friend, not just another person who will desert them if the mood takes me. From the very beginning of my outreach work, I was touched when people told me that it made them feel really important and appreciated that I would talk to them about my own problems or frustrations, that I valued their opinions and insights and treated them like fellow human beings.

Our mobile van was brilliant, but it only allowed DOTS to provide very basic street care, basic prescribing and treatment. We hit gold when a secret benefactor said that he would take it a step further and give us a fully functional veterinary vehicle. This was a huge step forwards, especially helpful in the winter and on rainy days. It was not only really important to have a clean, safe environment, but something we could use for every need we had. It was very clinical, it had a vet table, a blood-testing machine, and had running water and heating. It was just like walking into a very clean, sterile vet surgery with privacy for consultations, and an environment in which the dog's owner and the vet team could work together. It proved to be a huge success.

There was something about getting the proper van that made me reflect. For so long, I had thought that there was some Big Idea that I was close to finding, and I still did. Poppy was trying to tell me what it was. Everything so far had been brilliant and I was very proud of the achievements of DOTS – but, the aspect that still stuck in my throat was the fact that so many people on the streets had addictions and mental health issues that could be helped *if* they could take their dogs with them. I needed to move towards finding a place where they could stay together, a rehab centre for both. Dogs are the only constant in these people's lives and it's unbearably cruel to ask rough sleepers to give them up in order to help themselves get better.

As part of my ultimate dream, I knew what was next on the pathway to achieving my ultimate dream of a rehab centre – I envisaged a beautiful green space in the coun-tryside with boutique kennels for dogs who needed respite or foster care. They would be looked after as if they were superstars, loved and pampered, with access to all they could ever want.

I wanted to find somewhere that could become a sanctuary.

It would take a fortune. I began to think of as many fundraising campaigns as possible and I was filled with hope when people began to approach me to ask what they could do. DOTS was gaining a fantastic public profile and it meant that others wanted to help. *The Only Way is Essex* star, Pete Wicks, got in touch in 2019 and said he would do anything for us, anything at all. I knew he did a lot for animals, so I met him in East London, where we went for tapas and a drink. Eight hours later and we were sorted! Pete is our Ambassador and is unrelenting in his desire to raise awareness of the work that DOTS do. He now deals with the media as the face of DOTS. I hate all of the PR stuff, but Pete is brilliant at that side of things. He'll do anything we ask, from bungee jumps to going to schools and educating kids about being a dog owner.

We had a 10K walk around Hyde Park and supporters ran marathons. We developed a new hashtag #dogswith-nopostcode. We now had a bank of twenty volunteers for The Strand, many of whom had been there from the start. There is a documentaries being made about DOTS that will be shown in cinemas across the whole of the UK. Peter Egan became an Ambassador, as did Anna Webb. Candice Brown, who won *The Great British Bake Off*, also came on board as an Ambassador, said that she would do all she could, helping at the station, baking cakes and going with Pete on school trips as she used to be a teacher.

Pete and I came up with the fundraising idea of doing a sleepout just to show people how hard it was. On a Friday night in 2019, in freezing temperatures, our film crew, our back office team, and our clinical director joined the two of us in rolling out our sleeping bags and mats, with huge bits of cardboard on already cold and damp ground to make beds for the night. Nothing more to protect us – and nothing to prepare us for a night of shivering hell. As the temperature dropped through the night, and the cold and frost fell down on our already shaking bodies, our faces and hands were gripped with numbness.

The ground became even more damp and ice appeared on the surface of what should have been protecting and keeping us warm, our sleeping bags. We all tossed and turned, letting out words of despair as we realised there was no way of getting comfortable and warm, to get what was vitally needed to help us function – a good night's sleep. No hot drinks to warm us, nothing, just that sleeping bag, a roll mat and cardboard to keep us alive. The little sleep the team got, and the getting up and walking about to ensure there was feeling in the feet and body, was exhausting. There was no respite.

We woke from an unsettled night to birds singing and sirens blaring around us. It was 5.30 a.m. but we were silent with tiredness. It was eerie as we packed up. It had hit us hard, first-hand, what our homeless community, both with and without dogs, endure every night they spend out on the streets. The stiffness in our backs, the numbness of our hands and feet and faces, the relief that we survived, will never be forgotten. The only comfort the team got was from each other. Tonight, we are all in the warm, but tonight they roll back out their sleeping bags, lay the cardboard out, and snuggle up with their dogs to hopefully survive to fight another day. I have always tried to live my life by the maxim that you never look down on someone unless you are helping them up, and after that night, I realised just how worthy every soul on the street truly is.

The fundraising paid off and finally, on 2 January 2020, the day arrived – and what an amazing day it was. We had found our new home – The Sanctuary. Everything I had ever dreamed of had come true: three acres of peaceful green land, 64 kennels, four bedrooms for staff, plus a separate one-bedroom flat, a swimming pool for the doggies, and plans for a vet practice.

Over the next two months, I paused to reflect on what I'd achieved so far. I couldn't believe it all really. Three years ago, I'd launched that first station on The Strand and hoped that maybe two or three dogs would turn up if I was lucky. Now I saw about thirty every Sunday and knew of hundreds more across the UK, either via our station, hubs or outreaches. It had taken a team of incredible people and it warmed my heart to know that there were such generous souls out there.

But my reflection wasn't the only thing that started in early 2020 – coronavirus had hit the world, and everything was about to be turned on its head. By April, things were going on as close to normal as possible – but normal had changed so much. People were starting to wear masks, there were daily government announcements warning us to stay at home, save lives, protect the NHS. For street people, none of that was relevant to them in any way. They couldn't choose to stay at home, they couldn't choose what would happen to them, but decisions were being made behind the scenes that would impact on them a great deal.

The station at The Strand continued as it was – as always, it proved to be the biggest point of need. Vet care, however, had to be emergency only and was as vital as ever, but the social side, the interaction with the street homeless and their dogs, had to be scaled back enormously. There was simply nothing we could do about this. It was an epidemic, the likes of which had never been seen in our lifetime and we just had to adapt as best we could.

I had to keep myself and my team as safe as possible. We delivered food to locations where it could be collected as the dogs still needed regular and healthy diets wherever possible; I didn't want to turn the clock back on all the good work we'd done in that area and have the dogs overweight and filled with poor food again.

The Sanctuary went into lockdown for humans unless they were onsite staff and the numbers of dogs on the street that needed access to us increased as Westminster City Council decided to clear the streets. Rough sleepers were offered temporary accommodation – but without their beloved dogs. That's where DOTS stepped in.

The homeless were basically decanted from the streets, with their dogs – as always – not allowed to follow. It was an emergency situation for everyone, and I had to just accept it rather than argue that they shouldn't be separated. This was a fight I had had so many times and, if I couldn't manage to change so many minds about it when things were 'normal', I'd have no chance now. It was better that we got involved so that they weren't both on the streets – human and dog – but it was the same old problem. Our volunteers simply couldn't self-isolate through this period, and I'll always be in awe of their courage and the fact that they put themselves at risk in order to help the dogs and people we work with.

I had to work with as many pathways and support services across the UK as humanly possible. I also opened up The Sanctuary to NHS workers who needed places for their dogs as it was so important to do our bit for the heroes who were taking care of all the sick. If NHS staff lived alone and were worried about their canine companions, I wanted to do all I could to help. These amazing frontline workers were keeping our country together, which meant that opening up The Sanctuary for them was the least I could do. This allowed them to work and rest without worry about that part of their life and I was glad I could do it.

I also reached out to the London Ambulance Service so that any dog-owning patient with suspected or positive COVID-19 going into hospital could be reassured that we would collect and care for their dog at The Sanctuary. They'd know it was loved and nurtured, not in a bare kennel somewhere.

Sadly, we ourselves were never considered key workers – not me, our vets, our vet nurses, our frontline volunteers, all of whom put our lives on the line from the start through that difficult time. Like many, we had to beg for contributions of PPE, such as masks, gloves, and hand sanitiser. Times were hard and donations were down a huge amount – but times have been hard for me before. However, this time, there was the added worry of COVID-19, which I was believed to have contracted. I had never in my life felt so bad. I was completely whacked out, unable to even raise my head from the pillow for weeks on end. I have a respiratory problem, so I guess I was always in the at-risk group, but I never considered just hiding away. There was always someone in a worse position than me, and I had to just get on with things.

I pulled through. I always have. I had been doubted by so many people. I had been told I was mad to even think of doing this with a charity that was only thirty-three months old. I was put down, told I had taken on too much and that an idea like The Sanctuary would be too big for me to handle, that it would never work. Well, to all those who doubted me – you gave me strength, you gave me the courage to succeed. To all those who believed in me, helped me on those days I felt like giving up, who gave me hope and encouragement, you gave me the power to focus on the future when I took hold of the keys of The Sanctuary.

Some days I think 'God, look what I've done!' and then other days I think 'God, what *have* I done?' It's a bit of a rollercoaster, overwhelming at times. In many ways it's scarier now than back then as more people need us and it's getting harder to keep generating the resources we need. Back then, I had no idea of what I would grow, how huge it would become. It's a bit like working on the same wavelength and mindset of a homeless person actually – I try to think of the here and now. We don't know what tomorrow brings, yesterday has been. You can't plan anything with street sleepers; you can't say, 'I'll meet you two o'clock Thursday' because it will never happen if they don't know the time or the day. At The Sanctuary, I might need to have more awareness of diaries and calendars but I still have to think of what is required just in that very moment.

When you tell your story, you heal. Everyone's life is tricky at times – we all face trauma and loss. We grieve because we love, that's just the deal. However, we also have to find a way of getting through, of navigating. Poppy taught me that. Difficult times make us who we are. Homeless folk know this more than most and I am amazed at what they cope with. Working with them is not without cost and I take on their trauma, which means that I need a way to process it all. Thankfully, writing Poppy's story – our story – has helped me share the truths of our journey together. I always knew she'd changed me and left a remarkable legacy. I didn't know just how much until I put it all down on paper.

I can't deny that I'm shedding a tear as I write this. I miss her so much. I wish she was sitting beside me at the laptop, nudging me, licking me, wanting to be tickled and kissed, smiling her Staffie smile. I ache for Poppy sometimes; I do wish I'd had her for longer, but I also bless the time we did have together. I know she'll be waiting for me at Rainbow Bridge, but until then, all I can do is think of her and say . . .

Who would ever have thought one little street dog could inspire so much? Who would ever have thought you would be the making of me and save all of those other lives too? Who would ever have thought you would have an impact that will last forever?

Thank you Poppy, thank you my darling girl.

I'll see you again one day and we'll be together forever –
Mummy xx

Credits

Michelle Clark and Seven Dials would like to thank everyone at Orion who worked on the publication of *Poppy the Street Dog*.

Editorial
Marleigh Price

Copy editor
Clare Wallis

Proof reader
Loma Halden

Audio
Paul Stark
Amber Bates

Contracts
Anne Goddard
Paul Bulos
Jake Alderson

Design
Rachael Lancaster
Joanna Ridley
Nick May

Editorial Management
Jane Hughes
Alice Davis

Finance
Jasdip Nandra
Afeera Ahmed
Elizabeth Beaumont
Sue Baker

Marketing
Brittany Sankey

Production
Katie Horrocks

Publicity
Kate Moreton

Sales
Laura Fletcher
Esther Waters
Victoria Laws
Rachael Hum
Ellie Kyrke-Smith
Frances Doyle
Georgina Cutler

Operations
Jo Jacobs
Sharon Willis
Lisa Pryde
Lucy Brem